Also by Peter Greenberg

The Travel Detective

Hotel Secrets from the Travel Detective

The Travel Detective Flight Crew Confidential

The Traveler's Diet

The Traveler's Diet

Eating Right and
Staying Fit on the Road

Peter Greenberg

VILLARD 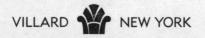 NEW YORK

No book can replace the diagnostic expertise and medical advice of a trusted physician. Please be certain to consult with your doctor before making any decisions that affect your health, particularly if you suffer from any medical condition or have any symptom that may require treatment.

A Villard Books Trade Paperback Original

To my mother, who was always on my case
about my weight . . . and was always right.

And to all the travelers and road warriors
who know that, in the end, less is more.

Contents

The Traveler's Diet

CHAPTER 1

Diet Another Day

The last time I weighed what I was supposed to weigh was in 1969. I remember it well. It was New Year's Eve, and that was the night I gave up smoking.

Three days later, I was in Israel, on the border with Syria, covering a continuing border war. We were in foxholes, and someone had launched mortars toward the Israeli positions. As the explosions came way too close for comfort, the other journalists with me were convinced we were going to die.

Suddenly, behind me, two Israeli soldiers appeared, and were handing out disgusting French cigarettes. Two of the other journalists, guys who had never smoked, accepted them and lit up. When the soldiers got to me, I attempted to decline politely, saying I was "trying to quit." The war seemed to stop for about fifteen seconds while everyone looked at me incredulously, as if to say, "You're trying to quit? We're all about to die anyway. Take the cigarette!"

I didn't. We lived. And I haven't had a cigarette since. OK, so much for the good news.

But from the morning of January 6, 1970, when I returned home, I was on Oreo patrol. Snack food. Junk food. You name it, I went for it. And it showed. If it's true that you are what you . . . overeat, then I was the *pie* piper.

I became obsessed with certain "foods." I had an obscene relationship with Diet Pepsi, drinking up to twenty cans a day. I found a candy connection online, in McKeesport, Pennsylvania, and ordered those red Swedish fish candies in bulk. I didn't just stop there: Around my office you'd always find peanut M&M's, Snickers, and Root Beer Barrels.

In 1987, I went on a serious diet supervised by a doctor, and I lost 51 pounds. Then I started traveling for *Good Morning America* for seven years, and the weight came right back—and then some.

Despite all good intentions, no matter what shape you're in, or whatever your exercise program, travel is the great enemy. The minute you leave home, your routine takes an immediate vacation. And as more and more people travel, it's becoming obvious that obesity is no longer an American disease. It has become a global pandemic. And as obesity rates soar, so has diabetes. In 1985, diabetes afflicted 30 million people worldwide. A little more than a decade later, that figure had escalated to 135 million. The good news—one could argue—is that as you are reading this, about 100 million Americans are on a diet. The bad news: Our lifestyles, coupled with our increased travel schedule, work against us winning the weight war.

And it shows. I was never overweight as a kid. I didn't eat a lot of junk food in high school, but that's when I discovered Linden's chocolate chip cookies in the cafeteria. By the time I became an executive at Paramount, they were delivering chocolate chip cookies to the office.

I love snacking. And snacks were everywhere. There were potato chips and popcorn in the office, pretzels and peanuts on the plane, chocolates waiting in my hotel room when I arrived. Let's not talk about the minibar. And we haven't even gotten to the social breakfasts, lunches, and dinners that go along with the job.

I hate scales. Always have. My mother, the queen of the less-than-subtle hint, gifted me each Christmas with a beautifully wrapped . . . scale. After the first year (this went on for more than ten years), I stopped opening the "present."

Dostoyevsky once wrote that every man lies to himself. At the very least, we're in serious denial when it comes to diet and exercise. I fooled myself into thinking that, given my lack of serious food vices—and all things being relative, my excess weight was an acceptable trade-off.

Apparently, I wasn't alone. More than 30 percent of adults in America are obese, and the number who are overweight has tripled in the last twenty years. We are addicted to junk food, and, worse, our national food supply is the number one source of chronic disease.

I fit perfectly into some pretty scary statistics, many related directly to my travel schedule. A friend once told me that you should never eat anything served to you out of a window unless you're a seagull. And yet, the odds that an American will eat at a fast-food restaurant on any given day are one in four. Well, I did better than that. Three out of four days, you could find me at an airport, or in a rental car on assignment on the road, pulling off the highway long enough to get supersized. And on that fourth, fifth, sixth, and seventh day? I was eating out, at a hotel or a restaurant. Again, I was in trouble: That hotel or restaurant meal was 170 percent *larger* than a meal prepared at home. Odds that a person will closely follow a diet are, again, one in four. That was me as well (I was one of the other three). Then there were statistics that were not even close to describing me: The amount the average American spends annually on candy is $84. (I was spending at least ten times that amount.)

As the son of a doctor, and with my travel schedule, I get a checkup once every three months. The results, despite my weight, have never been cause for alarm. Blood pressure was always a little high, and triglycerides and cholesterol were always high but not out of control. I hadn't smoked in more than thirty years; I hardly drink alcohol. Don't drink coffee.

When I went to see Raymond Keller, a brilliant and talented physician, in March 2005, for another checkup, I thought that once again I could just breeze right through. He had always told me to lose weight and limit my intake of sweets and junk food, and, of course, I never listened.

But on this visit, the numbers started to catch up with me. My blood pressure was 145/95, and the cholesterol and triglyceride numbers were frightening. Then it was time to stand on the scale. I was more than a little embarrassed. I knew I weighed too much, but nothing prepared me for the number that confronted me. I weighed in at a whopping 284 pounds.

I thought: I can't control the weather. I can't control the political situation, and I can't control who's driving on the freeways. But I *can* control what I eat and how much I put in my mouth.

I knew I had to do something about this, but where to start?

Each week there are at least three new diet books published. I was confronted with a little bit of everything: Actually, I was confronted with more than I could digest (every pun intended).

- 3-Hour Diet

- 6-Day Body Makeover

- Abs Diet

- Atkins Diet

- Blood Type Diet

- Cabbage Soup Diet

- Jenny Craig

- Curves

- Fat Flush Plan

- Fit for Life

- French Women's Diet

- Glycemic Index

- Grapefruit Diet

- Bob Greene

- Hamptons Diet

- LA Weight Loss

- NutriSystem

- Dr. Phil

- Perricone Promise

- Scarsdale Diet

- Slim-Fast

- South Beach Diet

- Step Diet

- Sugar Busters

- WeightWatchers

- The Zone Diet

There was even an eat-all-the-bread-you want-for-life diet!

To challenge me more, I felt I had two strikes against me: no discipline and no guidance. And that was quickly counterbalanced by . . . shame.

That night, I had dinner with my editor at *Men's Health*, Stephen Perrine. I told him of my disappointing checkup and that I was now motivated to lose weight. "But you travel more than anyone else I know," he said. "How can you possibly stick to a diet and exercise program?" The problem, of course, is that so many of us travel, that on any given day even the most well-intentioned diets are jettisoned, timetables and discipline evaporate . . . And therein was the genesis of this book. Could we develop a diet and exercise plan that worked not only at home, but on the road, given all the obstacles? It was worth a try.

Like any good traveler, I needed a road map. First, Perrine made me keep a food diary for a week. And when I was finished with it, it didn't make for pretty reading.

Without realizing it, I had become the poster child for the Nabisco telethon—Chips Ahoy!, Fig Newtons, and the real killers, Wheat Thins. Entire boxes would be consumed at a single sitting . . .

A typical seven days in my life from early 2005:

MONDAY

6 A.M.	Awake
	No formal breakfast
	Diet Pepsi
	Three chocolate chip cookies
8 A.M.	Two Red Delicious Apples
8:30 A.M.	Diet Pepsi
10 A.M.	Six pieces of cherry Swedish fish
11 A.M.	Another Diet Pepsi (keep in mind, I never finish one—just about three hits per can)
12:30 P.M.	Lunch: sushi
4 P.M.	Red Delicious Apple
6 P.M.	Popcorn
8:30 P.M.	Dinner: Thai food—beef, pork, chicken satay, mee krob (crispy sweet noodles)
11 P.M.	Red Delicious Apple
	And yes, a few more Swedish fish

TUESDAY

Same waking time
Same morning habit
Lunch: skirt steak and sautéed string beans
Same afternoon habit
But no dinner. Instead, the red-eye to Chicago
(On the plane, no meal—but generous helpings of
    mixed nuts and, of course, Diet Pepsi)

WEDNESDAY

5:30 A.M.   Arrive
Bagel and cream cheese
Diet Pepsi/Coke
Lunch: cheeseburger (no fries)
No dessert

4 P.M.   Arrive at hotel
Here's where problems start. The hotel has sent up
chocolate-covered strawberries, cheese, crackers, et al.,
    and they are devoured by yours truly.

8 P.M.   Dinner at hotel restaurant: rack of lamb, no dessert
Late night: chocolate-covered peanuts (ugh) and, of
    course, some Diet Pepsi

THURSDAY

No breakfast (there's a pattern here)
Early morning ride to the airport
At the airport, a Snickers bar
On the plane, cereal and milk for breakfast, and the
    ritual Diet Pepsi lunch in L.A.: sushi
3 P.M.   Snacking on Swedish fish
6 P.M.   Popcorn
9:30 P.M.   Late Thai dinner

And back at the house: I devour a full bag of pistachio nuts.

I'm an idiot!

FRIDAY

Early flight to San Francisco

Bagel and cream cheese at the airport

Working lunch at meeting: roast beef sandwich, potato chips, Diet Coke, and cookies

Back to L.A. (peanuts on plane)

Dinner at deli: pastrami and swiss on rye with Russian dressing

Late night: chocolate-covered almonds

SATURDAY

Early morning Diet Pepsi ritual

Red Delicious Apple

Tape television show: cookies, honey-roasted nuts, and licorice on the set

4 P.M.   Flight to New York: steak on plane (disgusting) and Diet Pepsi

Midnight   Arrive in New York

I probably left out a lot of guerilla-raid snacking, and that week included only one hotel. It could have been worse. It was a thoroughly embarassing diet, coupled with little or no exercise.

Once I handed in the food diary, I was already negotiating. For the new diet protocols, I asked to be able to keep four Red Delicious Apples a day (something I had been doing since I was a child) and at least a few Diet Pepsis.

Next stop was a nutritionist. Heidi Skolnik, a contributor to *Men's Health* and a friend, volunteered to help. Then Perrine arranged a meeting with an amazing trainer, Annette Lang. The only non negotiable: I had to listen to them, and I couldn't cheat.

Team Greenberg was formed. And before long, others were added, including dieticians, food researchers, scientists, sleep experts, chefs, and other trainers from around the world. What we've done in this book is look at every single possible component part of the travel experience as it relates to diet, exercise, sleep, time zones, and all the other absurdities, anxieties, and imponderables of the travel world. From that, we developed and then embraced a lifestyle, and a discipline, that allowed me— and now you—to either stay in shape or lose weight, or both, at home and on the road.

Was it easy? Of course not. I travel 400,000 miles a year. Was it worth it? Absolutely. And believe me, if I can do it with that travel schedule, anyone can do it.

CHAPTER 2

Before You Leave: Preparing for the Worst-Case Scenario

Between two evils, I always pick the one
I never tried before.

—Mae West

This is not a book about eating or traveling healthy. This is more about eating and traveling healthier, and perhaps most important, it's about eating and traveling smart. That's not often easy, considering that anytime you travel, the odds are against you. Plans are soon abandoned or changed. In the end, your schedule is only something to depart from. And your regular patterns are disrupted. You've got to adjust, or you're a diet and exercise victim before you ever leave home.

First, some statistics. A 2003 study done by the American Dietetic Association and ConAgra Foods revealed these facts:

- Six out of ten Americans plan to take one to two trips each spring and summer, and three out of ten plan to take three to four trips.

- Thirty-two percent of travelers are more likely to pack food or snacks from home for their trips than a year ago.

- When traveling with children, 65 percent say they are more likely to bring food or snacks from home.

- Nearly all (97 percent) of those driving to their vacation destinations will pack a meal for the road.

No surprises there, but you need to think about how long you will be traveling. Then account for delays and multiply by two. Will you need snacks along the way? Of course you will. Do you really want to eat airline food? Of course you don't. Have you built time in for walking? Do you have the exercise equipment you'll need on the road? Or access to it?

"There are two kinds of overweight people," my friend James Boyce likes to say. "They are overweight because of hereditary problems, and it's horrible, or they're overweight because they're not taking care of themselves, and that's unforgivable."

And Boyce should know. When I first met him, the award-winning chef (now cooking at the Montage Resort in Laguna Beach, California) weighed in at 320 pounds. He now weighs a healthier 185. He is my idol: He's a chef and he lost the weight. What was my excuse?

According to Boyce, it's not so much *what* you eat as *how much* you eat. "Unless you have serious allergies," he says, "the reality is that you shouldn't cut everything out that you like because it will never work in the long run. It's OK to have potatoes and bread and butter, but you need to limit your intake and then exercise appropriately." Boyce cooks with butter. He eats well, and he managed to lose more than 130 pounds doing just that.

Thus, as I began to create a food and exercise protocol, I only asked for certain accommodations. I knew this would be a radical adjustment to my lifestyle, but as Heidi, Annette, and others developed my road map, I asked to be able to keep my regimen of four Red Delicious Apples a day and at least a few Diet Pepsis. And one day a week, a thick, greasy cheeseburger. I would no longer be in denial, but every once in a while, I wouldn't be denied.

Some other new rules:

- A whole new approach to what—if anything—I eat at airports and on airplanes.

- At every hotel I visit, minibars will be either locked or removed. Reason: Who needs the temptation to add the unnecessary and unhealthy calories?

- When I check in, I will not be escorted to my room, but to the fitness/health center. If we're honest with ourselves, then we'll realize that we don't really change our lifestyle when we change our location. Left to our own devices, we'll go right to those devices—literally—and in my case, if I'm allowed to bypass the gym, I'll go right to the . . . BlackBerry.

- Here's the tough one: Wherever and whenever possible, no main meal eating after 8 P.M.

Part of the new regime is simply about preparation and taking a three-pronged approach to diet, exercise, and sleep. That preparation starts at home, before you ever travel anywhere.

And that's where Heidi Skolnik kicked in. Skolnik, among other things, is the sports nutrition consultant to the New York Giants and the School of American Ballet. (Already I'm feeling better!) She is also a nutritionist at the Women's Sports Medicine Center at the Hospital for Special Surgery.

"The key for travelers," she explains, "is to create structure in an unstructured world. And that's often so hard . . . but it's not impossible."

So Heidi created a special program for me. It started with some general advice:

- Drink one cup of water per hour on the plane. (I can also substitute juice, tea, seltzer, tomato juice, or the like.)

- Choose soda (diet) no more than twice a day, preferably with food.

- Call ahead and have a salad, fruit and yogurt, an omelet, or hard-boiled eggs waiting for me upon arrival at my hotel.

- *Do not* get the key for the minibar.

- Do get an apple or an orange to keep in my room for the morning.

- Work out in the morning before I fly whenever possible. Take a walk when I get to my destination if time allows, especially if it is daylight.

- While on the flight, get up and walk the aisle or stretch my legs every ninety minutes.

- Expect the unexpected. Expect delays. Buy or bring snacks and food along to the airport and on the plane (Au Bon Pain salad and/or fruit yogurt parfait, GroveStand apricots and nuts, Nature Valley Granola Bar).

Now, for specifics.

THE GREENBERG PLAN

"You have to anticipate change in your schedule as much as possible," Heidi Skolnik argues. "This means looking ahead in the day and anticipating when your three meals and snacks will be—even if this means eating in a taxi while going cross town to a meeting."

In my particular case, she looked specifically at my schedule and determined that I was already sabotaging myself. "You scheduled your day so tightly you forgot about *you* in there," she pointed out. The key is to schedule a workout when you land and then go to a business dinner. Just say you are available at eight instead of seven-thirty or seven o'clock if that means getting your workout in, or, conversely, let your business meeting know you must be done by a certain time to make another commitment you have (with yourself, for a meal or a workout—they do not need to know what your next commitment is).

Then came the toughie: Begin to pay attention to how hungry you are before you eat and how full you get once you are eating. Match food with hunger. (More on this later.)

And finally . . . no more than the two Diet Pepsis a day, and always with food.

Skolnik put me on a 2,200-calorie-a-day diet, which broke down as follows:

Protein (25 percent)   137 grams
Fat (24 percent)   59 grams
Carbs (51 percent)   280 grams

	Starch	Veggie	Fruit	Dairy	Fat	Protein
	12 servings per day	4+ servings per day	3 servings per day	3 servings per day	59 grams per day	10 servings per day
Breakfast	2		1	1	10	2
Snack	1			1	10	
Lunch	3	2	1	1	10	3
Dinner	4	2			10	5
Snack	2		1		10	

Breakfast

	Starch	Veggie	Fruit	Dairy	Fat	Protein
	12 servings per day	4+ servings per day	3 servings per day	3 servings per day	59 grams per day	10 servings per day
Breakfast	2		1	1	10	2

Starch: Choose two of the following (in any combination: one each of two different choices or two of the same).

³/₄ cup cereal	1 pancake	¹/₃ of a bagel
¹/₂ cup oatmeal	¹/₂ English muffin	¹/₄ cup Grape-Nuts
1 tablespoon syrup	2 (4-inch) rice cakes	1 slice bread*
1 tablespoon jam/jelly	1 frozen waffle	¹/₂ doughnut
3 graham crackers	1 yogurt (lite) or ¹/₂ of a regular Dannon	

*Choose whole grain when possible.

Fruit: Choose one of the following.

1 piece	1/2 cup juice	2 tablespoons raisins
8 dried apricots	1/4 cup dried fruit	1 1/4 cup berries

Dairy: Choose one of the following.

1 cup (1 percent) milk (if choosing chocolate milk, count as one
    starch)
1 cup sugar-free yogurt (if regular Dannon, count also as two
    starches; if Stonyfield Farm, count also as one starch)

Fat: Choose up to two of the following.

6 nuts: almonds or cashews	1 tablespoon cream cheese
1 pat (teaspoon) butter	1 slice bacon
1 slice cheese	2 teaspoons peanut butter
10 nuts: peanuts	1 tablespoon seeds: pumpkin or sunflower

Protein: Choose two of the following.

1 egg or 2 egg whites	1 1/2 slices of cheese (or 1 ounce)
1 slice Canadian bacon	1 ounce lox
1/4 cup cottage cheese	(1 sausage link, 1 to 2 times per week)

Sample Breakfast Menus

2 pancakes	2 eggs	1/2 bagel with
1 1/4 cup berries	English muffin with	2 tablespoons
2 pats (teaspoons) butter	2 pats (teaspoons) peanut butter	cream cheese
2 slices Canadian bacon	1 cup 1 percent milk	2 ounces lox
1 cup 1 percent milk	Banana	6 ounces orange juice (or an orange or mixed berries)
		1 cup sugar-free yogurt

1 cup oatmeal	2 eggs
1/4 cup dried fruit	1 slice bacon
12 almonds or cashews	2 slices whole wheat bread or whole grain English muffin
2 egg whites with 1 ounce cheese	1 pat (teaspoon) butter
1 cup 1 percent milk or sugar-free yogurt	6 ounces orange juice

Lunch

	Starch	Veggie	Fruit	Dairy	Fat	Protein
	12 servings per day	4+ servings per day	3 servings per day	3 servings per day	59 grams per day	10 servings per day
Lunch	3	2	1	1	10	3

Starch: Choose three of the following (in any combination: one each of three different choices or three of the same).

1/3 of a bagel	1/2 cup oatmeal	1/2 pita
2 (4-inch) rice cakes	1 slice bread*	1 granola bar
1/2 cup corn	1/2 cup rice	1/2 cup pasta
3 graham crackers	1/2 cup of beans	3/4 ounce pretzels

1 yogurt (lite) or 1/2 of a regular Dannon
12 to 18 potato chips (add 10 fat grams)
1 tortilla (a wrap can be the equivalent of 3 to 4 slices of bread!)
About 20 tortilla chips (add 5 to 10 grams fat)
1 small potato (or sweet potato)
12 french fries (add 5 grams fat)
Sushi: 1 roll = 1 to 2 starches
1 slice pizza = 2 or more (depends on whether it's Domino's or a New York slice!)

3/4 cup cereal	1 pancake	1/3 of a bagel
1/2 cup oatmeal	1/2 English muffin	1/4 cup Grape-Nuts

1 tablespoon syrup	2 (4-inch) rice cakes	1 slice bread*
1 tablespoon jam/jelly	1 frozen waffle	1/2 doughnut

*Choose whole grain when possible.

If choosing an energy bar or candy, recognize that 15 grams of carbohydrate = one starch and incorporate accordingly.

Vegetable: Choose two of the following.

1/2 cup cooked   1 cup raw

Fruit: Choose one. (Remember: You can have more fruit and less starch.)

1 piece	1/2 cup juice	2 tablespoons raisins
8 dried apricots	1/4 cup dried fruit	1 1/4 cup berries

Dairy: Choose one of the following.

1 cup 1 percent milk (if choosing chocolate milk, count as one starch)

1 cup sugar-free yogurt (if regular Dannon, count also as two starches; if Stonyfield Farm, count also as one starch)

Fat: Choose up to two of the following.

5 nuts	1 tablespoon salad dressings
1 slice cheese	2 tablespoons reduced-fat salad dressing
1 pat (teaspoon) butter	1 tablespoon reduced-fat mayonnaise
1 teaspoon oil	1 teaspoon regular mayo
2 teaspoons peanut butter	2 tablespoons sour cream

Protein: Choose three of the following.

1 egg or 2 egg whites	1 1/2 slices of cheese (or 1 ounce)
1/4 cup cottage cheese	All meat by the ounce

Sample Lunch Menus

Tuna salad:
3 ounces tuna,
    drained and
    rinsed, with
    2 tablespoons low-
    fat mayonnaise
    and $1/4$ cup
    chopped celery
    ($1/4$ serving)
1 pita
2 slices tomato
    ($1/2$ serving)
1 large romaine
    lettuce leaf
 ($1/4$ serving)
1 cup carrot sticks
$1/2$ can canned
    pineapple

3 ounces sliced
    turkey breast
1 slice cheese
2 slices whole wheat
    bread
1 teaspoon mustard
    (free food)
2 slices tomato
    ($1/2$ serving)
1 large romaine
    lettuce leaf
salad ($1/4$ serving):
    1 cup cucumber
        slices
    $1/4$ cup onion,
        diced
    2 tablespoons
        dressing,
        low-fat
1 medium apple
1 granola bar

3 ounces sliced
    chicken breast
    over salad with
    mixed vegetables
    and $1/2$ cup beans
1 medium banana
    with 1 teaspoon
    peanut butter
1 cup 1 percent milk
3 graham crackers

Minestrone with
    Parmesan cheese
3 ounces grilled salmon salad
    with 1 cup romaine lettuce
    and 1 cup mixed
    raw vegetables
    (tomato, cucumber, pepper,
    onion, etc.) and
    2 tablespoons reduced-fat
    salad dressing
1 small roll or $3/4$ oz pretzels
1 medium apple or other fruit

Omelet: 2 eggs, 1 ounce
    cheese, $1/4$ cup mushrooms,
    $1/4$ cup tomato, $1/4$ cup green
    peppers, $1/4$ cup onions
1 English muffin with
    1 tablespoon cream cheese
1 cup yogurt
1 cup mixed berries

Dinner

	Starch	Veggie	Fruit	Dairy	Fat	Protein
	12 servings per day	4+ servings per day	3 servings per day	3 servings per day	59 grams per day	10 servings per day
Dinner	4	2			10	5

Starch: Choose four of the following.

¹/₃ cup pasta	¹/₂ cup corn
¹/₃ cup brown rice, long-grain	³/₄ ounce pretzels
1 small potato (3 ounces)	¹/₂ cup beans and peas: garbanzo,
¹/₂ cup mashed potato	kidney, pinto, black-eyed
1 slice whole wheat bread	6 wheat crackers, fat-free
1 mini whole wheat bagel	¹/₂ cup lentils
¹/₂ English muffin	¹/₃ cup hummus
¹/₃ bagel	¹/₂ pita
2 (4-inch) rice cakes	1 small whole wheat roll

Veggie: Choose two of the following.

¹/₂ cup cooked	1 cup raw

Examples: Tomato, spinach, romaine lettuce, carrots, broccoli, celery, mushrooms, peppers, cauliflower, eggplant, zucchini, asparagus, onions, cucumbers, artichokes

Fat: Choose two of the following.

1 tablespoon mayonnaise, low-fat	1 teaspoon soft margarine
2 tablespoons salad dressing, low-fat	1 teaspoon oil
6 nuts: almonds or cashews	1 teaspoon butter
10 nuts: peanuts	¹/₂ tablespoon peanut butter
1 tablespoon seeds: pumpkin or sunflower	

Protein: Choose five of the following.

1 egg or 2 egg whites	3 ounces fish: cod, flounder,
3 ounces turkey breast	haddock, halibut, trout, lox
1 ounce lox	3 ounces chicken breast, white,
½ cup tuna, drained and rinsed	no skin

Sample Dinner Menus

5 ounces grilled fish
1 teaspoon lemon
  juice
1 cup brown rice
½ cup cooked
  spinach
½ cup mushrooms
  sautéed in
  2 teaspoons oil

Shrimp cocktail
1½ cup pasta
½ cup tomato
  sauce and
  broccoli
¼ cup fresh
  mushrooms,
  sliced
½ cup spinach
/₄ cup fresh carrots,
  grated
Parmesan
  cheese

Mixed green salad
5 ounces steak
  (sirloin, filet
  mignon, New York
  strip),
1½ cup mashed
  potatoes with
  2 tablespoons
  sour cream
1 cup cooked mixed
  vegetables
  (broccoli, carrots,
  green beans, etc.)
  with 1 teaspoon
  oil
1 small roll

5 ounces grilled chicken
½ cup black beans
1 cup Spanish rice
1 cup grilled vegetables
  (green peppers, red
  peppers, onion)
1 ounce grated cheese

4 ounces lean ground beef
  hamburger
1 ounce cheese
1 medium bun
2 slices tomato
1 large romaine lettuce leaf
1 slice onion
1 cup corn with 1 pat butter
½ cup cooked asparagus

Snacks

	Starch	Veggie	Fruit	Dairy	Fat	Protein
	12 servings per day	4+ servings per day	3 servings per day	3 servings per day	59 grams per day	10 servings per day
Snack A	1			1	10	

Starch: Choose one of the following.

⅓ cup pasta	½ cup corn
⅓ cup brown rice, long-grain	¾ ounce pretzels
1 small potato (3 ounces)	½ cup beans and peas:
½ cup mashed potato	garbanzo, kidney,
1 slice whole wheat bread	pinto, black-eyed
1 mini whole wheat bagel	6 wheat crackers, fat-free
½ English muffin	½ cup lentils
⅓ bagel	⅓ cup hummus
2 (4-inch) rice cakes	½ pita
	1 small whole wheat roll

Dairy: Choose one of the following.

1 cup fat-free milk
1 cup yogurt, fat-free, no added sugar
2 slices (1½ ounces) cheese, reduced-fat
½ cup cottage cheese, low-fat

Fat: Choose two of the following.

1 tablespoon mayonnaise, low-fat	1 teaspoon soft margarine
2 tablespoons salad dressing, low-fat	1 teaspoon oil
6 nuts: almonds or cashews	1 teaspoon butter
10 nuts: peanuts	½ tablespoon peanut butter
1 tablespoon seeds: pumpkin or sunflower	

Sample Snack A Menus

1 cup yogurt, fat-free, no
added sugar
¹/₄ cup Grape-Nuts
12 almonds

1 slice whole
wheat bread
1 tablespoon
peanut butter
1 cup 1 percent milk

	Starch	Veggie	Fruit	Dairy	Fat	Protein
	12 servings per day	4+ servings per day	3 servings per day	3 servings per day	59 grams per day	10 servings per day
Snack B	2		1		10	

Starch: Choose one of the following.

¹/₃ cup pasta
¹/₃ cup brown rice, long-grain
1 small potato (3 ounces)
¹/₂ cup mashed potato
1 slice whole wheat bread
1 mini whole wheat bagel
¹/₂ English muffin
¹/₃ bagel
2 (4-inch) rice cakes
¹/₂ cup oatmeal

¹/₂ cup corn
³/₄ ounce pretzels
¹/₂ cup beans and peas:
garbanzo, kidney, pinto,
black-eyed
6 wheat crackers, fat-free
¹/₂ cup lentils
¹/₃ cup hummus
¹/₂ pita
1 small whole
wheat roll

Fruit: Choose one of the following.

1 medium piece of fruit:
banana, apple, orange, etc.
¹/₂ cup juice
¹/₄ cup dried fruit
1³/₄ cup berries

Fat: Choose two of the following.

1 tablespoon mayonnaise, low-fat	1 teaspoon soft margarine
2 tablespoons salad dressing, low-fat	1 teaspoon oil
6 nuts: almonds or cashews	1 teaspoon butter
10 nuts: peanuts	$^{1}/_{2}$ tablespoon peanut butter
1 tablespoon seeds:	
pumpkin or	
sunflower	

Sample Snack B Menus

1 cup oatmeal with	4 rice cakes
$^{1}/_{4}$ cup dried fruit	1 tablespoon
2 tablespoons seeds	peanut butter
	1 banana

It wasn't easy, but I started. My biggest challenges: breakfast . . . and Diet Pepsi. I don't eat breakfast, and some would say I was addicted to Diet Pepsi. That's a definite double negative.

I started with breakfast, and cut down on the Diet Pepsi gradually until I eliminated diet soda entirely.

An amazing thing happened in the week following the elimination of the Diet Pepsi: I found myself falling asleep at eight o'clock each evening. I was actually coming down from the caffeine!

Then I embarked on a whole new water regimen. I took my current weight—about 284—and divided it in half. That's the number of ounces of water I began drinking each day—about 140 ounces, or seven 20-ounce bottles. I didn't think I could do it. But then I figured out a way to make it happen: I went out and bought smaller, 8-ounce bottles of water. Right by my desk, I kept a seventeen-bottle countdown list. I found I could polish off two of the small bottles every thirty minutes, and simply check off the list, bottle by bottle. So the breakfast (which filled me up in the morning), coupled with the water and the exercise, began to make a dent in my weight.

OK, all that might work at home, but what about on the road? And how would I really keep track of what I was doing when I was traveling?

ON THE ROAD AGAIN

Heidi Skolnik became my own personal portion-teller. She allowed me to have high-fat meat twice a week, but it all came down to portion size. Unless I were a seven-foot basketball center, a 20-ounce ribeye would be lethal. At Chinese restaurants, chicken with vegetables was acceptable, but orange chicken (fried) was verboten. And since I am partial to Asian food, Skolnik taught me a trick: Separate the food onto individual plates, leaving the sauce behind, then throw on extra vegetables to fill up the plate . . . and no refills. At Thai restaurants, I'm allowed pad thai only if I share the dish.

To keep me honest, Skolnik introduced me to an innovative new online system called Nutrax. It lets travelers use their camera phones to snap pictures of their meals and easily build a photo food log. But even without the camera, logging on to www.nutrax.com is an eye-opening experience. The concept, started in 2004 by Noah Knauf and Thomas Batten, let me log on anytime with my own food report. Let's say I entered into the system that I ate a chocolate chip cookie. The system would immediately ask what brand of cookie and how many. When I input my response, it instantaneously lists the calorie, fat, sodium, and carb content. You know right away if you're violating your allotted daily intake; the system alerts you if you are in trouble. It also works with PDAs, so it's perfect for road warriors.

What the Nutrax system doesn't account for is excuses, and when I first started the program, I was full of them.

Madelyn Fernstrom knows all about excuses. She hears them every day, as the founder and director of the Weight Management Center at the University of Pittsburgh Medical Center. She's spent the past twenty-five years studying and treating obesity and eating disorders.

I met Dr. Fernstrom one day in the greenroom for the *Today* show, and since people never hesitate to ask me for travel advice, I asked for hers. She described to me the five worst mistakes people who travel make when it comes to diet. According to Dr. Fernstrom, the first mistake is when people *eat to combat fatigue.* She explains: "They'll say 'I'm tired, so I'll eat something to give me energy.' And a typical selection," she reports, "is something high in sugar and high in fat. Now that's a terrible combination."

She told me about Donna, an Internet executive for a worldwide company, who travels about twenty days a month. "I'm always tired," she says. Noticing that her weight was creeping up to the tune of 5 pounds a month, she and Dr. Fernstrom took a look at her eating patterns. "I thought I was doing so much restaurant eating—that was the problem," Donna said. "But I have been following the lifestyle plan we agreed on." Probing a little further, it turned out that Donna was grazing at the airport between meals, for energy. With downtime of about an hour before a flight, Donna would try to revive her energy level by grabbing a Cinnabon with a coffee or a big, doughy pretzel with a diet soda. "I need the quick energy," she would rationalize.

Best solution: Donna started taking a 200-calorie energy bar for her airport layovers, and selects only diet soda or coffee with skim milk and low-cal sweetener. If she indulges at the airport between meals, she chooses a small frozen yogurt—nonfat and sugar-free—in a dish rather than a cone.

The second big mistake is the *basic lack of planning* for a plane trip. "People will argue that they were so busy that they missed lunch or dinner and as a result they were starving on the plane flight," Fernstrom reports. And therein lies the problem. When you're overhungry, everything looks good—even airline food—and that's when overeating occurs.

David, an attorney, has a hectic schedule, and often misses meals. On a travel day, he tries to pack in as many meetings as possible, and cuts it close at the airport. He found he was always running to the gate, leaving no time to eat. When he finally was able to sit down and eat on the plane, he would devour whatever was served. While flying in business class, he would vacuum up two dishes of nuts, have several extra rolls, and clean his plate. "I didn't realize I was so hungry," he explained.

One solution: David started carrying two apples in his brief-case to pull out at the gate, prior to boarding. The crunch was a great stress reliever and prevented him from being overhungry on the flight, allowing him better control.

Number three on the Fernstrom list: *disconnecting from a lifestyle plan because of travel.* ("I'll worry about it later—who cares?") Many of us who watch what we eat to lose or maintain weight often decide to disconnect from a plan because it seems like too much effort to make good choices while we're on the road. Rather than disconnect altogether and eat whatever is put in front of you, Dr. Fernstrom suggests the dieter's Plan B: Make a better food choice. Maybe not the best choice, but a better one. This allows you to keep a measure of control, and prevents you from packing on too many calories.

Carol always closely monitored her eating, and had maintained a stable weight. She came to Dr. Fernstrom looking for a better way to control her eating, since she observed that when she traveled—particularly by car—she would just lose it altogether. She commuted between Pittsburgh and Washington, D.C. (about four hours), spending her workweek in Pittsburgh and weekends in D.C. She acknowledged that she needed to keep her mouth busy during these long trips.

Best solution: Dr. Fernstrom suggested that she keep a number of "free" foods in the car for her commute—including sugarless gum, diet soda, and flavored low-cal water—and allow herself one treat when she stopped for gas, which would be a snack of her choosing for around 200 calories. This made room for the reward she was seeking to compensate for her long drive, yet it kept her in control. She also agreed to plan on having a meal either before or after the trip. Leaving right after a meal would help her avoid getting overhungry; knowing she would be eating as soon as she arrived would help her avoid temptation during the trip.

The fourth big mistake is what Dr. Fernstrom refers to as *Calorie-Clueless Syndrome:* the problem of *not* being aware of the calorie content of foods that you eat. Things that seem lower in calories because they contain less fat are the most common culprits. People will shun fast food, thinking it is poisonous for a dieter, yet they will blithely purchase an extra-large, doughy pretzel or an oversized turkey wrap because it is "healthy." Even worse is choosing trail mix filled with nuts and dried fruits—and packed with calories. A 6-ounce bag can have more than 1,000. Another major sabotage is the coffee kiosk. There's a big difference between a small latte (100 calories, sweetened with low-cal stuff) and a grande mocha latte (more than 300 calories). This is the time to admit that calories count. A great choice when selections are limited, either on a plane or on the road, is any kind of "kid's meal."

Best solution: John liked a "complete meal," and he didn't like to wait. Knowing that a kid's meal hamburger contains a total of around 500 calories—250 for the hamburger and 250 for the fries, with a Diet Coke—he could indulge in a modest caloric load for a low cost (particularly at airports!), with quick service. For him, this took the guesswork out of the caloric challenge.

Dr. Fernstrom also suggested that John purchase a fast-food calorie guide (available at all bookstores). John recognized his temperament, knew what he wanted to eat, and was willing to gather information.

The fifth and final big mistake that people make when watching their travel diets is failing to monitor *liquid calories*. This doesn't just mean alcohol—avoid *all* liquids (except skim milk). Juice, energy drinks, flavored waters, smoothies, mixed drinks—all of these can pack on a lot of calories. Read the labels, and don't waste calories on liquids. Not only are calories from alcohol weight promoting, but they make you more vulnerable to overeating because they sabotage your self-discipline.

Best solution: Barry cut out the "healthy" smoothie he felt he needed for plane trips by substituting a banana, which would give him the same sense of fullness without the calories of the banana blend—a whopping 300. On the plane he would allow himself one light beer for every two-hour flight, which accounted for most of his travel time. He would also have one bottle of water, in addition to the one bottle of beer. This plan helped him with his control—and with his confidence.

FINAL PREDEPARTURE TIPS

Here are some other things to consider before you head for the airport.

The Truth about Jet Lag

Some experts suggest that you preset your body clock in an attempt to prevent jet lag. I mention this only as a suggestion for people who are convinced they get jet lag. Some likewise recommend extravagant diets to prevent jet lag. I'm not a big fan of these anti–jet lag diets, which usually involve a complicated trade-off between feast and fast days before you travel. However, one of the most popular and well-respected ones is the Argonne Diet.

According to this program, you need to start three days prior to departure:

- Avoid alcohol. Although it may induce drowsiness initially, it results in a fragmented sleep.

- Avoid caffeine. It takes a few days to clear caffeine from your body. Do not consume caffeinated food or drinks within six hours of bedtime.

- Eat high-protein breakfasts and lunches.

- Eat high-carbohydrate dinners to bring on drowsiness through increased release of serotonin, which promotes sleep.

Two days prior to departure:

- Avoid alcohol and caffeine.

- Lower your caloric and carbohydrate consumption.

One day prior to departure:

- Repeat the regimen prescribed for three days prior to departure.

Day of departure:

- Fast, then determine a breakfast time at your destination. Sleep until this breakfast time, if possible.

- Eat a protein meal and remain awake after breakfast.

- Caffeine consumption in the morning is OK if you are traveling west (where your day will seem longer).

- Caffeine consumption in the evening is OK if you are traveling east (shortened day, heading through night).

Upon arrival:

- Eat meals at destination times rather than at the times you ate at your point of origin.

- Consume a high-protein lunch.

- A high-carbohydrate dinner will stimulate drowsiness (increasing serotonin release to promote sleep).

- Remain awake until your destination bedtime.

If you are unable to sleep at your destination, get out of bed, move to another area, and return to bed only when you feel sleepy. Bedtime relaxation routines, such as a warm bath, reading, and watching TV, signal the brain to prepare for sleep.

Acclimatize the next day.

I have some friends who insist they get jet lag flying between Los Angeles and San Francisco or between New York and Washington, D.C., but I hardly recommend such intense preparation for these short flights. In my particular case, I don't follow any of these predeparture routines for any flights, be they short shuttle hops or marathon runs such as a nonstop flight from New York to Singapore.

I dislike some of these anti–jet lag diets because they actually tell you to ingest caffeine before you are trying to go to sleep.

"There's very little evidence this works," says Timothy Monk, professor of psychiatry at the University of Pittsburgh Medical Center's Western Psychiatric Institute and Clinic. "Most of the success of these anti–jet lag diets is anecdotal, and the one study done was with "incredibly motivated folks who suffered very little jet lag anyway. It wasn't a fair test for a middle-aged traveler like myself."

My advice: Complicated anti–jet lag diets don't work. The time to fight jet lag—if you really think you're susceptible to it—is during and after travel, and we'll get to that in depth in a later chapter.

The key to trip preparation is basic common sense:

- Keep up your exercise routine so it's easier to maintain when you are on the road.

- Pack early.

- Don't eat spicy food or greasy hamburgers just before bedtime on the night before you travel.

- Drink lots of water, because you are going to get dehydrated on the plane.

- Get a good night's sleep!

In addition, try to schedule a flight that lands in your arrival city in the late afternoon or early evening so you won't have to stay up that long once you get there and can get a good night's sleep. If you arrive in the early morning after a long flight, you'll be more tempted to take a long nap when the rest of the folks back home are starting their days, and it will take you longer to adjust in your new time zone.

Many people will tell you that if you are traveling for business and are expected to perform, you should arrive a day early to allow your body to acclimate to its new surroundings. That sounds good, but on a practical level, it just never happens. Instead, try to schedule meetings for later in the morning, so that you are able to build in some time for moderate exercise before your business meetings.

Expect the Unexpected

Which usually means you'll be delayed. Research where you're going, including layover cities, so that you can make your unexpected delay useful. Explore the city or visit a museum. If you're stuck at the airport, take a walk.

Don't Leave Hungry

You know what it's like to go to the grocery store hungry. That's always a no-no. Make sure to eat a filling breakfast if you are flying in the daytime or a healthy dinner if you are flying overnight.

The hardest part of being a business traveler is not having time. If you are running from the office to the plane, grab something healthy at the airport (I'll tell you where in Chapter 3) before you get on the plane.

Brown-Bagging It

Whether you are traveling by train, plane, or automobile, the best way to control what you are eating on the road is to take it with you. So do what I do. Bring your own. In the past, I didn't plan ahead, and I ended up spending—or, I should say, *over-spending*—nearly $40 or $50 per trip buying stuff at the airport that I not only didn't need but really didn't want. Now I take along a six-pack of 8-ounce bottles of water and four apples. And believe it or not, that's it.

Dietician Cynthia Sass never gets on a flight without a meal replacement bar, nuts, and fruit. As I've mentioned, plenty of water is important to prevent dehydration as well. And finally, baby carrots or other raw veggies that you can eat with your hands are a convenient travel snack.

Sass recommends bringing nonperishable food on the plane. Why? "So much of the food people bring on planes actually raises the risk of foodborne illness," she says, "because people will often bring sandwiches and/or food they've purchased in the airport yet wait to eat." What this means is that perishable food could be in the danger zone—a temperature between 40°F and 140°F, at which bacteria grow rapidly. You can't see, smell, or taste a difference in food with a high bacteria count, so a sniff or taste test won't really tell you whether the food is OK.

Remember to wash your hands with soap and water during food preparation, especially between tasks. If you can't get to a restroom to wash your hands with soap and water, pack moist towelettes or a hand sanitizer to clean up before digging in. If you plan to cook family favorites like hamburgers, hot dogs, or chicken at home to take with you on your trip, remember to cook them to the proper temperatures: hamburgers to at least 160°F, hot dogs reheated to 160°F, and chicken to 170°F. Consider packing easy-to-transport, shelf-stable foods such as single-serve boxes of cereal, trail mix (but watch those calories!), popcorn, single-serve applesauce, cans of tuna, peanut butter sandwiches, fresh fruit, carrots, and celery.

The American Dietetic Association strongly recommends that you don't let food sit out unrefrigerated for more than two hours; in hot weather (above 90°F), the time is reduced to one hour. Here are some tips for handling perishable food:

• Pack food with a frozen ice pack or ice in an insulated lunch bag or cooler—and remember to drop in a refrigerator thermometer to ensure the temperature is kept below 40°F.

- In hot weather, transport food in a cooler (packed with ice or ice packs) in the backseat of an air-conditioned car instead of in the trunk.

- If you don't have access to a cooler, try packing frozen juice boxes or bottles of water for a hydrating refresher that will also help keep other foods around them cool.

Don't forget that carryout and fast food are also susceptible to food poisoning.

There's not much good to say about airline meals—on the carriers that still serve them, that is—but the one good thing about them is that they must adhere to strict safety standards in terms of their preparation.

You Can Take It with You: Workout Gear You Can Carry On

These days, you don't need an extra suitcase to take exercise gear with you. You'd be surprised what you can fit in your carry-on.

Workout Clothes
Quick-dry clothing that you can wash out in the sink at your hotel and hang to dry is a must. If you are going to a cold climate, think in terms of layering and fleece.

Shoes
Nobody likes to pack bulky running shoes, but at present there is still no light roll-up shoe on the market that provides the support of a traditional athletic shoe.

However, if you wear your athletic shoes on the plane—much less likely to set off the metal detector than dress shoes—you'll save space in your carry-on.

If walking is more your speed for exercise, fashion is now

your friend. Some of the trendiest styles, from Adidas to Vans, come in neutrals and other colors that look so much more stylish than plain white sneakers.

Make sure that the shoes you bring along are ones you've already broken in. The last thing you want is to travel with blisters.

Exercise Equipment

Once you've sussed out what your hotel has to offer, you'll know how much of your own equipment you'll need to bring along to sustain your workout. Here are some possibilities:

- *Inflatable weights.*   AquaBells are made of heavy-duty vinyl. Just fill them with water, for a weight of up to 32 pounds per pair ($49.95). They also have ankle weights you can attach with Velcro ($24.95). They are guaranteed not to leak. Deflated, the dumbbells weigh 24 ounces, while the ankle weights are a mere 8 ounces—small and light enough to pack in your briefcase. (www.aquabells.com)

- *Zura Fitness Swimming Kit.*   This portable kit includes an inflatable kickboard, an inflatable leg float, a mesh bag, and an absorbent swimmer's chamois (about $16). Zura doesn't have dealers in every state, but you can search for local stores at zura.com or you can purchase the kit on the Web.

- Exercise tubes and bands.   Designed for the traveler, the Travel Fit Kit ($14.95) includes two exercise bands in your choice of light/medium or medium-to-heavy resistance levels and a hotel room workout on CD with over twenty different exercises. The kit includes upper- and lower-body exercises as well as some for abdominal and lower back muscles. It also includes a travel pouch. One drawback is that it is not compatible with Macintosh computers, so beware. (www.healthytravelnetwork.com)

- SPRI PRX-R Pumping Rubber Workout Kit.   This package includes three Xertubes of varied resistance, along with a door attachment, which is good for the hotel room. It also includes a thirty-minute instructional video ($29.99). Available at Target and Amazon.com.

- Travel Yoga Mat.   Just over a pound, this mat is thin and light and easy to fold in your luggage. (www.matsmats mats.com)

- Fitness balls.   Another portable fitness prop that has become ever more popular is the exercise ball. The original use for these balls was in physical therapy, according to a survey by the IDEA Health & Fitness Association, the world's leading membership organization of health and fitness professionals. However, the use of fitness or stability balls at fitness clubs has increased from 35 percent in 1998 to 87 percent in 2005. They are especially good for building up your abdominal, back, and hip muscles. Using the ball makes it harder for you to balance in the movement you are performing, which means that your core muscles—or your whole body, depending on the exercise—must work together to remain stable.

   If you are 5 foot 7 inches or under, a 55-centimeter ball will work for you. If you are taller, you might want to buy the larger 65-centimeter ball. Exercise balls can cost anywhere from $15 to $60, but you can easily find them for about $20. For more about how to use these exercise balls as well as purchase information, contact Resist-a-Ball, Inc. (www

.resistaball.com). They are also available at Target, Wal-Mart, and many other stores.

Inspiration
And finally, here is some equipment to keep you motivated:

* *A portable CD player/radio.* The treadmill is a lot easier when you are walking to your favorite music. At 1½ ounces, the iPod nano couldn't be much lighter. (www.apple.com)

* *GPS fitness trainers.* If you don't want to count on an unreliable pedometer, try a GPS trainer ($160). Rather than measuring the length of your steps, a GPS trainer uses global positioning system signals from space to measure the distance you travel. Worn on the wrist, the Garmin Forerunner 201 tells you your precise speed, distance, and pace. It also provides a Virtual Partner as a training companion. Once you set your training pace and distance goal, your on-screen animated partner runs at your desired gait. Below him, you get a graphic perspective of yourself either falling behind, speeding ahead, or keeping pace, so you can always check your wrist to see whether you're keeping up. This device is capable of storing data from your exercise regimen using proprietary software to chart your progress, including how many calories you've burned during your workout. (www.garmin.com)

Before you pack anything, however, call your hotel. Many hotels now loan equipment—from yoga mats to skis—so before you go lugging your favorite gear along on your trip, check with the hotel. It's so much easier knowing that it's waiting for you at the other end.

Of course, all this gear means nothing if you don't know how to properly use it. And this is the toughest thing I had to learn—not just the concept and the discipline of exercise, but what to do, when to do it, and why. And that's where Annette Lang, my supertrainer enters the picture.

My first meeting with Annette, in a gym in midtown Manhattan, was, to say the least, humbling. First, she took my measurements:

Chest	50.25 inches
Right arm	15.25 inches
Left arm	15 inches
Smallest part of waist	51 inches
Hips	48.75 inches

That was embarrassing enough.

But then it was on to the treadmill, followed by lat pull-downs, leg curls, bridges on a stability ball, reverse crunches, straight-arm pulldowns, and shoulder presses. Impressed? Don't be. I was pathetic. I was breathing hard, and the entire workout lasted . . . eighteen minutes. Ugh!

We soon moved the program over to the gym at the New York Sheraton Hotel on 53rd Street, and then a few weeks later, to the Parker Meridien Hotel's gym, called Gravity. For the next year, whenever I was in New York, I put in three days per week in one of those two gyms, or three days a week in gyms around the world (see Chapter 6). These workouts averaged an intense sixty minutes at a time. But none of this could have properly prepared me for the real test in terms of exercise (and self-control) that was to come . . . the airport!

CHAPTER 3

At the Airport

Let's face facts. Airports are not basically conducive to health, exercise, or sanity. I am convinced that the people who design them have never had to use them. Airports are generally not people-friendly, but that can actually work in your favor if you understand this ahead of time. To compound matters, a move by most U.S. airlines in the past few years to end free meals on most domestic flights, combined with a sharp spike in air traffic and the fact that many fliers are arriving at the airport hours ahead of time, has caused more consumers to crowd restaurants, fast-food counters, and snack shops at just about every airport.

And that's not a good sign, unless you choose your food wisely.

At Denver International, for example, food and beverage sales jumped 18 percent in 2005. Translation: A lot of people are eating and drinking there, and there is a high likelihood that their choices are not healthy ones.

Sales at the three McDonald's franchises in Denver International Airport, for instance, rose 22 percent, and many of those passengers brought the food onto their flights. Trust me—health issues notwithstanding, few things smell less appetizing than a McDonald's bag about an hour into a flight inside an enclosed airplane cabin.

On the other hand, there's also been a spike in the number of airport grab-and-go meals that can be brought on planes. Often, these meals include premade, prepackaged sandwiches, salads, and other items. A healthy alternative, you say.

But therein lies a seductive trap.

The key to staying fit on the road is to be conscious of every opportunity to do something that's healthy for your body. Every step of the way presents either a danger or an opportunity. Considering the odds that your flight will be delayed or canceled, that extra time can wreak havoc with your dietary discipline. When you're a wait watcher (and when it comes to airports, I've spelled that term correctly), you're more inclined to eat, even when you're not hungry.

To me, airports used to represent a rotten combination of unnecessary punishment and unhealthy reward. First, there was the terrorism of just navigating through an airport, and then came the unhealthy reward: bad food.

Again, preparation is the key. If at all possible, eat before you get to the airport. There are a number of reasons for this.

There's eating because you're hungry. And there's eating because you think you earned the right. I have to admit to a past behavior pattern at airports that was, to put it mildly, sad. I would stand in a long security line watching Transportation Safety Administration agents strip-search nuns looking for tweezers, and as the wait got longer, I would begin to visualize my reward—a Mr. Goodbar, a pack of Twizzlers, a Big Mac. And when I finally got through the line, many times I would buy all three—that is, when I wasn't immediately seduced by the telltale aroma of . . . Cinnabon. Admit it, the smell is so tempting it's nearly impossible to resist.

For those of you who have succumbed (myself, once, included), here are some sobering numbers. The regular Cinnabon weighs in (deliberate choice of verbs) at a whopping 813 calories! I often joke that it's not a pastry, but a weapon.

If you think you are starving, think also about how that airport breakfast fits into your overall caloric intake for the day. If you pick up that Starbucks café mocha (400 calories) and blueberry scone (460 calories), that's almost 900 calories—a big chunk of your daily allotment. And if you think you'll save on calories by getting a plain bagel, think again—that baby packs 430 calories.

Let's just say that you're being smart and decide to bypass the mighty Cinnabon and snub the overpriced and calorie-loaded Starbucks. Instead, you think you'll be *really* smart and head for that turkey wrap. Prepare for a surprise: Vendors need to maintain the moisture content of that turkey wrap, especially since it could easily sit in the display window for some time, so many of them douse that sandwich in enough sauce to send the calorie count into the stratosphere—in some cases, equaling that Cinnabon.

Now here comes another surprise. They also sell a smaller Cinnabon, which tips the scale at just 339 calories. This could be a better choice for you, as absurd as that might seem.

Let us now return to that lowly bagel—not to praise it but to bury its reputation as a healthy alternative. I always thought—mistakenly, as it turns out—that a bagel with either light cream cheese or no cream cheese would serve as a satisfying substitute for a high-calorie airline meal. Then Jayne Hurley, a nutritionist for the Center for Science in the Public Interest, set me straight. "The aura of a bagel being healthy got going about ten years ago," she says, "but it couldn't be further from the truth. Eating a bagel is like eating five slices of Wonderbread."

Best bet: Keep moving until you see a concession that sells fresh fruit or yogurt. My nutrionist, Heidi Skolnik, says her favorite airport foods come from Au Bon Pain—sandwiches, salads, or yogurt with fruit (and/or a whole grain roll). She also recommends Wolfgang Puck salads and GroveStand nuts and dried fruits.

If there's an Au Bon Pain at your terminal, try the small fruit cup, for just 70 calories (no saturated fat or cholesterol) or the small strawberry yogurt with granola, for 310 calories. But beware of portion size. A large blueberry yogurt with fruit and granola will hit you with 620 calories and 13 grams of fat!

GET THERE EARLY AND DO SOME LAPS

Let's be honest. You're not going to burn too many calories sitting on that plane for hours, but one way to reduce stress and make sure you build exercise into your day is to arrive at the airport early and get in some extra laps.

The benefits of getting to the airport early are many. You can pass through security without being stressed—Or, more accurately considering most airport security, stressed *less*. Giving yourself an extra hour to walk will go a long way toward meeting your exercise goal for the day. And let's face it: As a result of draconian security procedures and people-unfriendly airport design, you're going to walk whether you want to or not.

For example, one of my most unfavorite airports, Miami International, is great for the long march. Recently, I landed in the new American Terminal D, where I had to go through customs and then connect to a flight in Terminal C. Total distance: 1 mile! And that was while schlepping luggage.

Walking will also help you get past that seductive Cinnabon smell, bypass the familiar odor of McDonald's, and head toward more healthy airport food to take with you on the plane.

FIND A SALAD IN THE FAST-FOOD AISLE

As planes have cut back on serving food, airports are filling the void. And, more often than not, they are filling that void with calorie-laden comfort food.

Madelyn Fernstrom says that the main worry for travelers is fatigue. "People eat for energy. As something to perk them up." The problem for travelers is that when you are stressed and tired, you tend to pick what's more palatable, and that translates into two bad words in the world of diet: *sweet* and *fatty*. Her advice: "Even if you're at Subway or McDonald's, get a grilled chicken salad or a kid's meal where the portions will be smaller."

It's hard to think of McDonald's as nutritious, but if you can't pass up the Golden Arches, you can at least get a kid's meal containing Chicken McNuggets (six pieces), Apple Dippers with Low Fat Caramel Dip, and an Apple Juice Box (6.75 fluid ounces) for a total of 440 calories and 16 grams of fat. Or, if you have your heart set on a hamburger, you can get a Double Hamburger, Apple Dippers with Low Fat Caramel Dip, and Apple Juice Box for 550 calories and 17 grams of fat. If you add cheese, however, the meal increases to 650 calories and 24 grams of fat. A better choice would be the Caesar Salad with Grilled Chicken for 220 calories and 10 grams of fat. Add 1.5 ounces of Newman's Own Low Fat Balsamic Vinaigrette and you'll add only 40 calories and 3 grams of fat, but choose the 2-ounce package of Newman's Own Creamy Caesar, and you just added 190 calories and 18 grams of fat.

When it comes to the rumor that a burger is better than a salad laden with creamy dressing, nutritionist Jayne Hurley has no patience. "I'm so sick of everyone saying the burger is better than the salad. There is no salad ever born that is going to clog your arteries like a burger. Always."

As a fast-food outlet, Subway offers many good choices. The Turkey Breast Deli sandwich has just 210 calories and 3.5 grams of fat. Subway's Roast Beef Deli sandwich has only 220 calories and 4.5 grams of fat. But beware the Tuna Deli, with 350 calories and 18 grams of fat, and the Chicken and Bacon sandwich that has 530 calories and 25 grams of fat. However, almost all of Subway's salads are under 200 calories, and if you choose their fat-free Italian dressing, 2 ounces will cost you only 35 calories, as opposed to 200 calories for the ranch dressing.

Another good rule of thumb is to simply avoid deep-fried foods at all costs. In the past, I made the mistake of thinking that Chinese food at the airport was healthier than McDonald's. I remember waiting for one late-night flight, and there I was, standing in front of that Chinese food outlet, Panda Express, justifying the Orange Flavored Chicken. It sure looked good, but it is deep-fried, which means it's about 480 calories and 21 grams of fat. If you get the same size serving (about 5.5 ounces) of Black Pepper Chicken instead, it will cost you only 180 calories and 10 grams of fat. If you're feeling even more virtuous, try the Mixed Vegetables, for just 70 calories and 3 grams of fat. And remember, if you add a serving of steamed rice (330 calories, 0 grams of fat), you'll exceed 800 calories if you pair it with Orange Flavored Chicken but consume just 400 calories if you choose the vegetables.

Also keep in mind portion size. If you stick with one entrée and rice, you have a meal, but indulge in two or three and you put a serious dent in your calorie allotment for the day.

NUTRITIONAL COMPARISONS

I asked dietician Cynthia Sass to come up with these comparisons of typical airport food, which might upend your expectations.

Comparison ☹	☺
Drinks Starbucks Java Chip Frappuccino® Blended Coffee Grande:	Starbucks Espresso Frappuccino® Blended Coffee Grande:
510 calories	230 calories
22 grams fat	3 grams fat
15 grams saturated fat	2 grams saturated fat
73 grams carbohydrate	46 grams carbohydrate
59 grams sugar	38 grams sugar
7 grams protein	5 grams protein
McDonald's Large Coke:	McDonald's Large Iced Tea:
310 calories	0 calories
0 grams fat	0 grams fat
0 grams saturated fat	0 grams saturated fat
86 grams carbohydrate	1 gram carbohydrate
86 grams sugar	0 grams sugar
0 grams protein	0 grams protein

Sandwiches

Au Bon Pain Chicken
  Mozzarella Sandwich:
740 calories
24 grams fat
4.5 grams saturated fat

73 grams carbohydrate
3 grams sugar
55 grams protein

Au Bon Pain Chicken
  Salsa Wrap:
440 calories
8 grams fat
1.5 grams saturated
  fat

68 grams carbohydrate
3 grams sugar
29 grams protein

Burger King Original
  Chicken Sandwich:
560 calories
28 grams fat
6 grams saturated fat

52 grams carbohydrate
5 grams sugar
25 grams protein

Burger King 5-Piece
  Chicken Tenders:
210 calories
12 grams fat
3.5 grams saturated
  fat

13 grams carbohydrate
0 grams sugar
14 grams protein

McDonald's Filet-O-Fish:

400 calories
18 grams fat
4 grams saturated fat

42 grams carbohydrate
8 grams sugar
14 grams protein

McDonald's
  Hamburger:
260 calories
9 grams fat
3.5 grams saturated
  fat

33 grams carbohydrate
7 grams sugar
13 grams protein

Subway Chicken & Bacon
  Ranch Wrap:
440 calories
27 grams fat
10 grams saturated fat

Subway Turkey Breast
  Wrap:
190 calories
6 grams fat
1 gram saturated fat

18 grams carbohydrate	18 grams carbohydrate
1 gram sugar	2 grams sugar
41 grams protein	24 grams protein

Salads

Wendy's Chicken BLT Salad with Honey Mustard Dressing:	Wendy's Mandarin Chicken Salad, no Crispy Noodles, with Oriental Sesame Dressing:
680 calories	433 calories
46 grams fat	24 grams fat
13 grams saturated fat	3 grams saturated fat
32 grams carbohydrate	43 grams carbohydrate
16 grams sugar	33 grams sugar (much from mandarin oranges)
37 grams protein	28 grams protein

Au Bon Pain Chicken Caesar Salad:	Au Bon Pain Mediterranean Chicken Salad:
530 calories	290 calories
22 grams fat	16 grams fat
10 grams saturated fat	4 grams saturated fat
40 grams carbohydrate	14 grams carbohydrate
1 gram sugar	2 grams sugar
41 grams protein	24 grams protein

Other

Taco Bell Regular Style Fiesta Taco Salad:	Taco Bell Fresco Style Ranchero Chicken Tacos (2):
870 calories	340 calories
47 grams fat	8 grams fat
16 grams saturated fat	2 grams saturated fat

80 grams carbohydrate	40 grams carbohydrate
10 grams sugar	4 grams sugar
31 grams protein	24 grams protein

Snacks

Starbucks White Chocolate Macadamia Nut Cookie:	Starbucks Shortbread Cookie:
470 calories	100 calories
27 grams fat	6 grams fat
8 grams saturated fat	3 grams saturated fat
54 grams carbohydrate	12 grams carbohydrate
34 grams sugar	4 grams sugar
6 grams protein	1 gram protein

Au Bon Pain Fruit Sours:	Au Bon Pain Large Fruit Cup:
400 calories	140 calories
0 gram fat	1 gram fat
0 gram saturated fat	0 gram saturated fat
105 grams carbohydrate	32 grams carbohydrate
91 grams sugar	30 grams sugar (natural)
0 grams protein	2 grams protein

While it might be hard to eyeball which sandwich has fewer calories, many chain restaurants, from Starbucks to McDonald's, post their nutritional information online. McDonald's has even announced plans to put nutritional information on its food wrappers (although one could argue that receiving nutritional information after you've bought the food is a little late).

Michael Jacobson, executive director of the Center for Science in the Public Interest, a nonprofit food-safety and nutrition watchdog group that supports legislation to put nutritional information on menu boards in New York and Washington,

D.C., gives credit to McDonald's for making this information public, but wishes that McDonald's would distinguish saturated and trans fat from total fat on its labels—an important distinction that he says would help Americans reduce their risk of heart disease.

He notes that McDonald's fried foods are high in saturated and trans fats because their potatoes, chicken, and fish are fried in a partially hydrogenated oil blend. A few years ago, McDonald's promised to reduce, then eliminate, trans fat in its cooking oils, but they have reneged on that promise, reportedly due to cost.

HEALTHY CHOICES

The good news, however, is that at most airports, contrary to popular belief, it is possible to get a good meal—to consume on the premises or take with you on the plane.

The Physicians Committee for Responsible Medicine also did some major investigative work for this book—at airports. The PCRM usually publishes an annual survey on airport food, but I asked them to expand their work for this book to include vendors and food selections from twenty-two different airports.

Chicago O'Hare International Airport flies high in first place this year, with a score of 92 percent, rising from fourth place last year and the bottom of the list in 2002. Phoenix Sky Harbor International Airport is this year's most improved airport, with a score that rose from 44 percent last year to 75 percent in the current survey. But Las Vegas's McCarran International, while improving nine points from last year, still sits on the tarmac with the lowest score, 42 percent.

In their annual survey, the PCRM nutritionists evaluated the restaurants in fourteen of the nation's busiest airports, giving each restaurant a point if its menu included at least one low-fat, high-fiber, cholesterol-free vegetarian entrée. The final percentage score was derived by dividing the airport's number of health-conscious restaurants by the total number of restaurants.

Airport	Score
1. Chicago O'Hare	92%
2. Detroit Metropolitan	89%
3. San Francisco	88%
4. New York	83%
5. Dallas–Fort Worth	81%
6. Denver	78%
7. Atlanta	77%
8. Orlando	76%
9. Newark	75%
10. Phoenix	75%
11. Los Angeles	69%
12. Minneapolis–St. Paul	68%
13. Houston	46%
14. Las Vegas	42%

But even the top-rated airports have significant room for improvement. Some airports have no more than a single healthy food choice, and more variety would be good. The best choices are low-fat and vegetarian.

Susan Levin, staff dietician for the PCRM, helped conduct and compile research for the Airport Food Survey. She says they were looking for dishes low in cholesterol and saturated fat. "We call these places and ask what they have easily available, not what the cook is willing to make. Something that is on the menu, easy to make. On the go," she reports.

Burger King offers a veggie burger, and if you're on a diet, it's worth the calorie savings. You can look at the nutritional value of various Burger King products online at www.bk.com and you'll see that a BK Veggie Burger has 420 calories and 16 grams of fat, but only 340 calories and 8 grams of fat if you hold the mayo. Compare that to an Original Whopper with cheese at a whopping 800 calories and 49 grams of fat.

Levin says that looking for vegetarian food without the cheese is one shortcut to healthy eating. "When you choose a vegetarian option, you are not getting as much of the saturated fat and [it is] lower in cholesterol, and it doesn't matter if you are vegetarian or not, those are the triggers for heart disease and obesity." When you order food, instead of asking, "Is that high in saturated fat or cholesterol?" you simply choose vegetarian. Levin advises that you look at the big picture when you're ordering. "If you can do a salad without the cheese and ranch dressing, it's probably going to be relatively low in calories."

Levin believes that what is driving the move for airports to make healthy options available is demand. "There's no other reason that people do anything other than to make more money. If people are demanding healthy food, people are going to provide it."

For this book, the PCRM expanded their search by individual airport and vendor. Here are their suggestions for healthy meals at airports around the United States.

Atlanta

- Atlanta Bread Company (Atrium): veggie sandwiches (hold the cheese and mayo); fruit salad; house salad; garden vegetable soup

- Au Bon Pain (Concourses B, D): vegetarian sandwich; garden vegetable soup

- Burger King (Concourses A, D): BK Veggie Burger (hold the mayo)

- Charley's Steakery (Concourses B, C): Veggie Deluxe sandwich (hold the cheese); garden salad

- Chili's Bar & Bites (Concourse D): black bean burger

- Chili's Too (Concourse A): black bean burger

- Great Wraps (Concourse A): veggie wrap (hold the cheese); black bean burrito (hold the cheese)

- Houlihan's (Concourse A, Atrium): veggie burger; Asian vegetable salad

- Le Petit Bistro (Concourse E): multiple vegetarian salads

- Manchu Wok (Concourse A, Atrium): Golden Plate (rice, vegetables, mixed vegetables); mixed vegetables

- Mandarin Express (Concourse B, E): vegetable lo mein

- Miller Lite Victory Lane (Concourse C): vegetable sandwich; garden salad

- Paschal's Southern Delights (Concourse A, C, Atrium): garden salad; vegetable plate (black-eyed peas, green beans, cabbage)

- Sbarro (Concourse B): spaghetti with marinara sauce

- Sports Scene (Concourse B): fruit salad; green salad; vegetable sandwich

- TGI Friday's (Concourse B): Gardenburger; garden salad

- Wall Street Deli (Concourse A): veggie sandwich (hold the cheese)

Boston

- Au Bon Pain (Terminal A, B, C, E): garden salad; veggie sandwiches made to order

- Bella Boston (Terminal B): pasta with marinara sauce; veggie club sandwich (hold the cheese)

- Boston Deli (Terminal B): make your own vegetarian sandwich or wrap

- Burger King (Terminals B, C): BK Veggie Burger (hold the mayo)

- Dine Boston Café (Terminal E): veggie wrap; vegetarian chili; veggie pizza (hold the cheese)

- Dine Boston Restaurant & Bar (Terminal E): vegetarian pizza (hold the cheese); grilled vegetable wrap (order without coleslaw and cottage cheese)

- Famous Famiglia (Terminal A): garden salad; spaghetti with marinara sauce

- Fox Sports Sky Box and Grill (Terminal B): no healthy items; unhealthy items include buffalo wings, nachos, BBQ pork sandwich, bacon cheddar burger

- Fresh City (Terminal A): veggie wraps and salads

- Fuddrucker's (Terminal A): Gardenburger; garden salad
  You can find many "less healthy" options on the Fuddrucker's website, but since the menu varies by location, I can't be certain what they serve exactly at this airport location. According to the website, you can get burgers as big as

1 pound and specialty burger options include Three-Cheese, Bacon Cheddar, and Southwest (which has bacon, cheese, and guacamole). They also offer a Crispy "Works" chicken sandwich (fried chicken, bacon, and cheese).

- Greenleaf's Grille (Terminal C): grilled veggie sandwich

- Jasper White's Summer Shack (Terminal A): grilled portobello mushroom sandwich; salad

- Killian's Boston Pub (Terminal B): veggie burgers

- Legal Sea Foods (Terminal C): veggie wrap; Vegetarian Box with lo mein, tofu, and vegetables

- Lucky's (Terminal A): Italian panini (hold the cheese); spinach and tomato salad; baby green salad with asparagus and tomato

- Samuel Adams Pub (Terminal C): vegetarian burger, salad and soup

- Sbarro (Terminal B, E): spaghetti with marinara sauce

- Wok 'n Roll (Terminal E): mixed vegetables and tofu with rice

Chicago O'Hare

- Artist and Writer (Terminal 1): Roasted Vegetable on Herbed Focaccia sandwich; fruit bowl; vegetable tray

- Berghoff Café (Terminal 1): veggie pizza (hold the cheese); pasta salad; fruit salad

- Burrito Beach (Terminal 3): veggie burrito (hold the cheese); black bean and rice burrito (hold the cheese)

- Café Zoot (Terminal 1): veggie sandwich (hold the cheese); garden salad

- Chicago Bar and Grill (Terminal 3): portobello sandwich; Gardenburger

- Chili's (Terminal 1, 2, 3): dinner salad (hold the cheese); black bean patty can be substituted for any burger selection

- Fox Sports Sky Box (Terminal 2, 3): portobello sandwich (hold the cheese); Garden Burger (hold the cheese)

- Gold Coast Dogs (Terminal 3, 5): veggie burger (hold the mayo)

- Goose Island Brewing Company (Terminal 2): veggie sandwich

- Great American Bagel (Terminal 1, 3): veggie bagel sandwich; minestrone soup

- Lou Mitchell's Express (Terminal 5): hot or cold veggie wraps (hold the cheese)

- O'Brien's Restaurant and Bar (Terminal 3): veggie tortilla wrap; salad

- Panda Express (Terminal 1, 3): vegetable chow mein; vegetable steamed rice; spicy tofu

- Prairie Tap (Terminal 3): portobello sandwich on wheat bun (hold the cheese); garden green salad

- Saladworks (Terminal 1): garden salad; veggie wrap

- Vienna Beef Hot Dogs (Terminal 1, 2): veggie focaccia

- Wolfgang Puck (Terminal 1, 3): spinach salad (hold the cheese); grilled vegetable sandwich; veggie pizza (hold the cheese)

Cincinnati

- Bluegrass Brewing Company (Concourse C): veggie burger; salads

- Gas Light Baking Company (Concourse C, Terminal 2 Ticketing): vegetarian sandwiches

- Gold Star Chili (Concourse B): veggie chili
  Less healthy choices: anything made with the standard ground-beef Cincinnati chili, especially a regular cheese coney made with regular chili, hot dog, and cheese, or a regular three-, four-, or five-way (nutrient comparisons at www.goldstarchili.com)

- Great Steak & Potato Company (Concourse B): Veggie Delight sandwich (hold the cheese)
  Less healthy options: Super Steak Sandwich (includes steak and cheese); Ham Explosion Sandwich (includes ham and cheese)

- 360 Gourmet Burrito (Concourse B): Teriyaki Smoked Tofu Burrito

- Watson Bros. Brew Pub (Concourse A): portobello mushroom sandwich

- Wolfgang Puck (Concourse B): pizza (hold the cheese); tomato basil pasta

Cleveland

- Great American Bagel (Concourse C, D, Food Court): veggie bagel sandwich; garden salad; fruit salad

- Great Lakes Brewing Company (Concourse A): Mostly less healthy choices including roast beef and cheddar sandwich; Original Sub with ham salami, turkey breast, and provolone cheese; chef salad with turkey, ham, swiss & cheddar cheeses

- Home Turf (Concourse D): Mostly less healthy choices including chili cheese fries; potato skins; chicken Caesar salad; bacon cheeseburger

- Judy's Oasis: Great menu offers a wide variety of healthy Middle Eastern food. All vegetarian menu includes hummus, baba ghanouj, lentil salad. *Best bet for healthy food.*

- Manchu Wok (Food Court): Mixed Vegetables, Black Mushroom Tofu, Garlic Green Beans
  Less healthy choices: General Tso Chicken, Sweet and Sour Pork, Hunan Beef

- Max & Erma's (Concourse B, C): Garden Grill Sandwich (hold the cheese); Black Bean Rollups
  Less healthy options (not necessarily on airport's menu): Simple Turkey Club Sandwich (turkey, bacon, cheese); Fish and Chips; Southern Fried Chicken Salad (fried chicken, eggs, two types of cheese); Max's Best BBQ Ribs (full or half slab of ribs with onion rings and cole slaw)

- Tequileria Bar & Grille (Concourse C): fruit plate; Jicama Salad; Mango Salad

Dallas–Fort Worth

- Burger King (Terminal E): BK Veggie Burger (hold the mayo)

- Chili's Too (Terminal B, C): black bean burger

- Frullati Café & Bakery (Terminal B, C): grilled veggie sandwich (hold the cheese); cold veggie sandwich (hold the cheese)

- Harlon's BBQ Grill & Bar (Terminal B): veggie burger; baked potato

- Los Amigos (Terminal A): bean burrito (hold the cheese)

- Manchu Wok (Terminal A, C, E): mixed vegetables with rice; veggie noodles

- Sbarro (Terminal B): spaghetti with marinara sauce

- Subway (Terminal A): veggie sandwich

- Taco Bell Express (Terminal A, C, E): bean burrito (hold the cheese)

- TGI Friday's (Terminal A, D, E): Gardenburger, garden salad

Denver

- Cantina Grill Express (Concourse A, B, C, Terminal Level 6): veggie burrito (hold the cheese); veggie taco; beans and rice

- Chef Jimmy's Bistro and Spirits (Concourse A): vegetarian panini (hold the cheese)

- Colorado Sports Bar & Deli (Concourse B): portobello mushroom sandwich (hold the cheese)

- Cozzoli's Italian Specialties (Concourse C): spaghetti with marinara sauce; garden salad

- Creative Croissant (Terminal Level 5): Mother Earth sandwich on wheat, rye, or sourdough (hold the cheese)

- Itza Wrap! Itza Bowl! (Concourse B): Teriyaki Veggie (cabbage, carrots, and rice in teriyaki sauce) or Colorado Sunshine (veggies and avocado) wrap or bowl

- Lefty's Colorado Trails Bar and Grill (Concourse A): portobello mushroom sandwich; Gardenburger

- Lefty's Front Range Grille (Concourse C): portobello mushroom sandwich; Garden Burger

- Lefty's Mile High Grille (Concourse B): Gardenburger; veggie Philly sandwich (hold the cheese)

- Panda Express (Concourse A, Terminal Level 6): vegetable steamed rice; mixed vegetables

- Pour La France! Café (Concourse B, Terminal Level 6): portobello sandwich

- ¡Que Bueno! Mexican Grille (Concourse B): veggie taco (hold the cheese); bean burrito (hold the cheese)

- Quizno's (Concourse A, B): veggie sandwich (hold the cheese)

- Sara Lee Sandwich (Concourse B): veggie sandwich (hold the cheese and mayo)

- Steak Escape (Concourse B): veggie sandwich (hold the cheese); garden salad

- Taco Bell (Terminal Level 5): bean burrito (hold the cheese)

- Wolfgang Puck Express (Concourse B): vegetarian salads; spinach pizza (hold the cheese)

Detroit

- Budweiser Brewhouse (McNamara Terminal): veggie sandwich

- Burger King (McNamara Terminal): BK Veggie Burger (hold the mayo)

- Charley's Grilled Subs (McNamara Terminal): Philly veggie sandwich (hold the cheese)

- Chili's Too (McNamara Terminal): black bean burger

- Mediterranean Grill (McNamara Terminal): tabbouleh; hummus; fattouch; stuffed grape leaves; vegetarian stir-fry; almond rice salad; Gardenburger

- Musashi (McNamara Terminal): veggie sushi, seaweed salad, tossed green salad

- National Coney Island (Smith Terminal): Greek salad; Gardenburger; veggie sandwich (hold the cheese)

- Online Café (McNamara Terminal): veggie burger

- Pasta Pasta (McNamara Terminal): veggie stir-fry with marinara sauce, garden salad

- PB & J (McNamara Terminal): gourmet peanut butter and jelly sandwiches

- Quizno's (Smith Terminal, McNamara Terminal): veggie sub

- Rio Wraps (McNamara Terminal): veggie wrap (hold the cheese)

- Sora Japanese Cuisine and Sushi (McNamara Terminal): veggie rolls; tofu rolls

- Taco Bell (McNamara Terminal): bean burrito (hold the cheese)

Houston

- Charley's Grilled Subs (E14): Grilled Veggie Delight

- Chili's (Terminal A South, B Gate Concourse): black bean burger

- El Paseo (Terminal A, North and South): taco salad (hold the cheese); bean burrito (hold the cheese)

- Famous Famiglia (E1): pasta with marinara sauce

- Panda Express (E1): veggie chow mein

- Pappasito's Cantina (E1): vegetable burrito (hold the cheese)

- Subway (Terminal C North, Terminal D Gate Concourse): veggie sandwich; salad

- Taco Bell (Terminal C, North and South): bean burrito (hold the cheese)

- Wendy's (Terminal C, North and South): baked potato (plain or with broccoli)

Las Vegas

- Big Apple Bagels: veggie sandwich; veggie salad

- Burger King (Terminal 1, 2): BK Veggie Burger (hold the mayo)

- Don Alejandro's Texan Grill (Terminal 1): vegetable burrito (hold the cheese)

- Jose Cuervo Tequileria (Terminal 1): bean burrito (hold the cheese)

- Port of Subs (Terminal 1): veggie sub

- Prickly Pear Bar & Grille (Terminal 1): veggie sandwich

- Quizno's (Terminal 1): veggie sub (hold the cheese)

- Ruby's Dinette (Terminal 1): Gardenburger

- Subway (Terminal 1): veggie sub

- Taco Bell (Terminal 1): bean burrito (hold the cheese)

- Wolfgang Puck Express (Terminal 1): veggie sandwich

Los Angeles

- Boudin Sourdough Bakery (Terminal 2, 7): veggie sandwich (hold the cheese)

- Chili's Too (Terminal 4): black bean burger

- Daily Grill (Terminal TBIT): pasta marinara; mixed green salad

- El Cholo Cantina (Terminal 5): beans with rice

- El Paseo (Terminal TBIT, 1): vegetable burrito, vegetable fajita

- Encounter Restaurant: grilled veggie sandwich; salads

- Hamada Orient Express (Terminal TBIT): vegetable chop suey; vegetable chow mein

- Java Java (Terminal 3, 6): veggie sandwich

- La Salsa (Terminal 7): bean burrito (hold the cheese); veggie tacos (hold the cheese)

- McDonald's (Terminal TBIT, 1, 5, 7): veggie burger

- Monet's, a California deli (Terminal 6): vegetable soup; veggie sandwich (hold the cheese)

- Ruby's Dinette (Terminal 6): vegwich (hold the cheese); veggie burger (hold the cheese)

- Sushi Boy (Terminal TBIT): udon noodles; vegetable sushi roll; vegetable combo (vegetable sushi roll and salad)

- Wolfgang Puck (Terminal 2, 7): veggie sandwich (hold the cheese); veggie pizza (hold the cheese); mixed greens salad

Manchester, New Hampshire

- Nutfield Pub and Café: Veggie Wrap (hold the cheese and cream cheese spread); fresh fruit platter at breakfast
  Less healthy choices: Breakfast Panini (with eggs, cheddar cheese, and bacon, ham, or sausage); Beer House Chili (ground

beef, topped with cheddar cheese and served with tortilla chips); French Dip Sandwich (roast beef and swiss cheese); BBQ Pork Sandwich

- Milltowne Grille: Boca Burger; Vegetarian Rollup (hold the sauce); Grilled Vegetable Pizza (hold the cheese); Grilled Vegetable Panini (hold the cheese and mayo)

   Less healthy choices: Muffaletta Panini (with ham, mortadella, salami, and provolone); Black Angus Bacon Cheeseburger; CBC sandwich (fried chicken breast, bacon, and cheddar cheese); Fish and Chips

Minneapolis

- Burger King (Main terminal, Concourse E, F): BK Veggie Burger (hold the mayo)

- California Pizza Kitchen (Concourse F): roasted veggie pizza (hold the cheese)

- Caribou Coffee (Concourse E, F, G): grilled portobello mushroom wrap

- Chili's To Go (Concourse G): black bean burger

- D'Amico & Sons Deli and Café (Main terminal, Concourse E): grilled veggie sandwich

- DQ Grill & Chill (Concourse C/D): vegetable sandwich

- Fletcher's Wharf (Humphrey Terminal): veggie sandwich (hold the cheese)

- French Meadow Bakery & Café (Concourse F): organic veggie made-to-order sandwiches

- Godfather's Pizza (Concourse A/B, C/D): veggie pizza (hold the cheese)

- Malibu Al's (Concourse C/D): veggie "lessadilla" (hold the cheese)

- Maui Taco (Concourse C/D): soft veggie tacos; vegetarian burritos (hold the cheese and sour cream)

- Quizno's (Concourse C/D): veggie sub (hold the cheese)

- Sbarro (Main Terminal, Concourse C/D, G): spaghetti with marinara sauce

- TGI Friday's (Concourse C/D): Gardenburger (hold the cheese and ranch dressing)

- Wok 'n Roll (Main Terminal, Concourse C/D): mixed vegetables; bean curd; veggie lo mein

Monterey, California
- Golden Tee Restaurant: veggie salad (hold the cheese)

New York—JFK
- Antonio's (Terminal 7): market greens salad; vegetable sandwich (hold the cheese)

- Atlantic Bar & Lounge (Terminal 7): roasted vegetable panini

- Away Café (Terminal 6): vegetarian sandwich

- Brooklyn Brew Pub (Terminal 1): roasted veggie sandwich (hold the cheese)

- Burger King (Terminal 3): BK Veggie Burger (hold the mayo)

- Carmela's Kitchen (Terminal 6): pasta and marinara

- Chili's Too (Terminal 3): house salad; black bean burger

- Cibo Express (Terminal 6): vegetarian wraps; salads

- Create Your Own Salad (Terminal 6): made-to-order salads

- Creative Croissant (Terminal 2): veggie sandwich (hold the cheese); garden salad; pasta salad

- Deep Blue Sushi (Terminal 6): veggie sushi, sautéed vegetables, seaweed salad, edamame

- Delancey's Bar (Terminal 4): Garden Burger

- Eurasia Coffee House (Terminal 1): roasted veggie sandwich (hold the cheese)

- Greenwich Village Bistro (Terminal 1): market greens salad; roasted veggie sandwich (hold the cheese)

- Latitude (Terminal 7): made-to-order salads; vegetable quesadilla (hold the cheese)

- McDonald's (Terminal 1, 4, 7, 8): veggie burger

- Mesa Picante (Terminal 4): vegetarian burritos; salads

- Mex and the City (Terminal 6): build-your-own veggie burrito

• Napa Valley Wine Bar (Terminal 1): roasted veggie sandwich (hold the cheese)

• New York Sports Grill (Terminal 6): veggie burger; salad

• Sbarro (Terminals 3, 4, 8): spaghetti with marinara sauce

• 7th Avenue Deli (Terminal 7): market greens salad; roasted vegetable panini

• Sky Asian Bistro (Terminal 6): Chinese vegetables; veggie fried rice; broccoli with garlic sauce; Buddha's Delight; veggie udon; spicy tofu

• Soup & KimBob (Terminal 1): grilled veggie sandwich; vegetable dumplings; garden salad (hold the cheese)

• Taste of the World (Terminal 4): Indian bean dishes; vegetarian Indian dishes; veggie lo mein

• Wok 'n Roll (Terminal 1, 2, 8): mixed vegetables; veggies and rice; tofu

New York — LaGuardia

• Akoya Sushi (Central Terminal): chilled edamame salad, seaweed salad, cucumber sushi roll, vegetable teriyaki entrée

• Anton's: Gardenburger (US Airways Terminal, US Airways Shuttle Terminal)

• Asian Chao (Central Terminal): tofu, vegetable lo mein

• Au Bon Pain (Central Terminal): veggie sandwiches made to order

- Brooklyn National Deli (Central Terminal): veggie sandwich; veggie wrap

- Coffee Beanery (Central Terminal; US Airways Terminal): grilled vegetable sandwich

- Cibo Express (Central Terminal): veggie sandwich; grilled veggie wrap; hummus and crackers

- Fox Bar & Restaurant (Delta Terminal): veggie burger; salad

- Jet Rock Bar & Grill (Central Terminal): Jet Rock Garden Salad

- Taco Bell (US Airways Terminal): bean burrito (hold the cheese)

Newark

- Asian Chao (Terminal B): tofu; mixed vegetables; vegetable soup

- Au Bon Pain (Terminal C): garden salad; gazpacho; veggie wrap

- Charley's Grilled Subs (Terminal B): grilled vegetable sandwich (hold the cheese)

- Chili's Too (Terminal B): black bean burger

- Famous Famiglia (Terminal A, C): pasta with marinara sauce; garden salad; fruit salad; cucumber/onion/tomato salad

- Formaggio's Café (Terminal C): veggie wrap (hold the cheese); Mediterranean salad (hold the cheese)

- Gallagher's Steak House (Terminal C): mixed green salad; baby spinach salad (hold the cheese); baked potato

- Garden State Deli (Terminal A): veggie sandwich (hold the cheese)

- Garden State Diner (Terminal C): pasta with tomato sauce; veggie burger; veggie salad

- Great Steak and Potato (Terminal A): veggie sandwich (hold the cheese)

- Greenleaf's Grille (Terminal A, C): veggie burger; veggie wraps; salads

- Le Petit Bistro (Terminal C): veggie sandwich; garden salad; rice and vegetables

- Maui Tacos (Terminal C): veggie burritos; veggie tacos

- Miami Subs & Grill (Terminal C): veggie wrap; garden salad; fruit salad

- O'Brien's Pub (Terminal B): veggie hoagie (hold the cheese); veggie stir-fry; veggie pasta

- Sarku (Terminal C): veggie lo mein; veggies with rice

- Vito's Gourmet Deli (Terminal C): veggie sandwich

- Wok 'n Roll (Terminal A, C): veggie lo mein; bean curd with veggies

Ontario

- Applebee's Grill: house salad; veggie burger

- California Speedway Café: veggie burger; veggie sandwich

- El Paseo: vegetarian burrito (hold the cheese)

- Jake's Bar & Deli: vegetarian sandwich (hold the cheese); garden salad

- Jake's Coffeehouse: vegetarian sandwich (hold the cheese); garden salad

- Round Table Pizza: vegetarian sandwich (hold the cheese); garden salad

Orlando

- Burger King (Gates 1–29, 60–99, HMS Marketplace): BK Veggie Burger

- Chili's Too (Main Terminal West Hall): black bean burger

- Fresh Attractions Deli (Main Terminal Food Court, Gates 60–99): gazpacho focaccia

- Macaroni Grill (Main Terminal): create-your-own pasta (red sauce, broccoli, onion, tomato, mushrooms, black olives, banana peppers)

- Miami Subs (Gates 30–59): garden salad; made-to-order veggie sandwich

- Outback Steakhouse (Gates 60–99): baked potato; garden salad; steamed vegetables

- Sbarro (Main Terminal): pasta with marinara sauce; (Gates 100–129): pasta with marinara

- Villa Pizza (Gates 30–59): pasta with marinara sauce; salad

- Zyng's Noodlery (Main Terminal): vegetable dumplings; spring rolls; Thai peanut noodles; Meal in a Bowl (choose rice or noodles, tofu, and vegetables); vegetarian Thai rice bowl; Vegetarian Zyng tossed Asian salad plate; vegetarian soup (rice or soba noodles, in Asian-flavored vegetable broth, with tofu, shiitake mushrooms, broccoli, corn, scallions, and cilantro sprigs); brown basmati rice and vegetables; tofu; zoya; lychees on the rocks for dessert

Phoenix

- Blue Burrito (Terminal 3, 4): veggie burrito (hold the cheese)

- Burger King (Terminal 4): BK Veggie Burger (hold the mayo)

- California Pizza Kitchen (Terminal 4): vegetable pizza (hold the cheese)

- Great Steak & Potato Company (Terminal 4): grilled veggie sandwich (hold the cheese); potato with veggies

- Kokopelli Deli (Terminal 3, 4): veggie sandwich

- Lefty's South Rim Bar and Grill (Terminal 2): veggie burger, baked potato

- Oaxaca (Terminal 4): veggie burrito; veggie taco salad

- Paradise Bakery & Café (Terminal 4): veggie sandwich (hold the cheese); fruit salad; green salad

- Sbarro (Terminal 3): spaghetti with marinara sauce

- Yoshi's Asian Grill (Terminal 4): veggie chow mein; avocado cucumber sushi

Richmond, Virginia

- Richmond Café Bar: portobello mushroom sandwich (hold the cheese)

Salt Lake City

- City Deli (International Terminal, Concourse B): veggie salad; veggie sandwich

- Great American Bagel (Concourse B): veggie bagel sandwich

- Sbarro (Terminal 2): spaghetti with marinara sauce; garden salad; tomato and cucumber salad

- Squatters Airport Pub (Concourse C): Buenos Dias Burrito (substitute tofu for eggs and hold the cheese); Squatters Breakfast Wrap (substitute tofu for eggs and hold the cheese); Grilled Veggie "Love Burger" (hold the cheese); Fresh Veggie Wrap (hold the cheese)

  Less healthy choices· Cobb Salad (chicken, bacon, two types of cheese, guacamole, tortilla chips, and ranch dressing); Pepperoni Pizza, Squatters Classic American Cheeseburger

- Terrace Restaurant and Lounge (Terminal 1): Terrace Salad, Tomato Basil Bruschetta

Less healthy choices: Chopped Cobb Salad (chicken, bacon, bleu cheese, eggs, and creamy dressing), Overstuffed Ham and Cheese sandwich

- Wall Street Deli (Concourse C): veggie sandwich; fresh fruit salad

San Francisco

- Anchor Brewing Company (Terminal 3): vegetable sandwich (hold the cheese)

- Andale Mexican Restaurant (Terminal 1, 3, International Terminal): veggie burrito (hold the cheese and sour cream); veggie tostada (hold the cheese and sour cream); vegetable Mexican sandwich

- Burger Joint (International Terminal): veggie burger

- Ebisu (International Terminal): udon noodles; ramen noodles; veggie sushi

- Emporio Rulli (International Terminal, Terminal 3): grilled eggplant sandwich (hold the cheese)

- Firewood Grill (International Terminal, Terminal 1, 3): fusilli marinara; mushroom pizza (hold the cheese); garden salad

- Fung Lum Express (International Terminal, Terminal 3): veggie soup; mixed vegetables; veggie chow mein; spinach with garlic sauce; braised tofu

- Harbor Village Kitchen (International Terminal): veggies and tofu rice plate; curried veggies and rice

- Jalapeno Taqueria (Terminal 3): veggie fajita (hold the cheese); veggie burrito (hold the cheese); rice and bean burrito

- Klein's Deli & Coffee Bar (Terminal 1, 3): garden salad; three-bean salad

- Lori's Diner International (International Terminal, Terminal 1, 3): veggie burger

- Osho Japanese Cuisine (International Terminal): vegetable sushi

- San Francisco Soup Company (Terminal 3): smoky split pea soup; daily special vegetarian soups; mixed greens salad

- Sankaku (Terminal 1, 3): veggie sushi; Teriyaki Tofu Bowl; Vegetarian Curry

- Tomokazu Japanese Cuisine: mixed vegetables; seaweed salad; vegetable sushi

- Willow Street Wood-Fired Pizza (International Terminal): veggie sandwich (hold the cheese); roasted vegetable pizza (hold the cheese)

Savannah, Georgia

- Budweiser Brewhouse: house salad

- Burger King: BK Veggie Burger (hold the mayo)

- Phillips Famous Seafood: house salad

- Southern Grill: house salad

Springfield-Branson, Missouri
- Airport café and lounge: garden salad and Boca Burger

Washington-Dulles
- Euro Café (Concourse A): salad; pasta primavera

- Ranch 1 (Concourse A): Gourmet Greens salad

- Sam's Brewhouse (Concourse B, D): Gardenburger

- TGI Friday's (Concourse D): Gardenburger

- Villa Pizza (Concourse B): pizza (hold the cheese); spaghetti with marinara sauce

And there's even some good news at smaller airports, where my previous experience was limited to guessing the age and pedigree of the mystery hot dog in the rotisserie.

Bozeman, Montana
- Overland Express: vegetarian salads (hold the cheese)

Charleston, West Virginia
- Gino's Pizzeria & Pub: spaghetti with tomato sauce

Grand Rapids, Michigan
- Home Turf Sports Grill: veggie burger

One airport that really stands out is Detroit's Metropolitan International, which has teamed up with the local Henry Ford Heart & Vascular Institute to provide more than fifty heart-healthy dishes at thirteen restaurants in the new McNamara Terminal. The best news: After the Wayne County Airport partnered with the institute, concessions increased 32.7 percent (from 2003 to 2004), and airport officials believe that the Heart

Smart program is partially responsible. The project has been so successful that it is expanding to the older Smith terminal, where they will be adding Heart Smart menu choices at eight additional existing restaurants.

BYOW

Before you get on the plane, make sure you have your own supply of bottled water. We'll talk more about airline water in the next chapter, but trust me when I tell you to bring your own.

While you're in the airport, avoid drinking alcohol. In addition to adding extra calories that you don't need—most drinks average about 200 calories and specialty drinks like piña coladas can have more than 300 calories—they'll also cloud your judgment, making it more likely that you'll splurge and consume those chips they serve with the drinks. Furthermore, drinking alcohol before you fly will contribute to your becoming even more dehydrated while you're on the plane.

So, if your plane has been delayed or you are experiencing the layover from hell, what do you do? Unfortunately, most of us simply eat—out of boredom. We sit there, we wait, and we watch other people wait. And we wait some more. Before long, we begin to feel that we simply *must* eat. But you don't have to feed your face. Instead, this is the time for some diversionary action. And believe it or not, at a growing number of airports, you can find it.

AIRPORT SPAS

Spas have begun popping up in airports around the country— perfect for massaging out those coach kinks, soothing tired skin, and refreshing travelers for the road ahead. The best part of this indulgence: no calories.

Here are some of the airports that currently offer spa services.

Baltimore-Washington International Airport

There are two Destination Relaxations, a chair kiosk on Pier B and a store on Pier D, which offer back, foot, and hand massages. (http://destination-relax.com)

Boston Logan International Airport

The Jetsetter Mini Spa is located on the departure level of Concourse C. A ten-minute massage is $15, a first-class manicure is $30, a coach manicure is $25, and an express facial is $30. The Jetsetter Mini Spa has another location at the Miami International Airport Main Terminal. (www.jetsetterspa.com)

Chicago O'Hare International Airport

The BackRub Hub in Terminal 3 offers back and neck massages (open 9 A.M. to 9 P.M.).

The O'Hare Hilton also offers massages and a full-service health club. A thirty-minute Swedish massage runs $50. (O'Hare Hilton: 773-686-8000)

Denver International Airport

A Massage Inc. services two locations in this airport, on Concourse A and on the mezzanine level of Concourse B. Frequent fliers can grab a haircut or a back massage. (303-317-0185)

Detroit Metropolitan International Airport

The OraOxygen Spa near Gate A45 offers oxygen treatments that run $18 for a fifteen-minute session. A thirty-minute massage is $45. (http://oraoxygen.net)

Indianapolis International Airport

The Passport Travel Spa, located in the Main Terminal, offers treatments such as a ten-minute Fast Track Manicure for $15 and a fifteen-minute chair massage for $18. (317-240-1050; www.passportnails.com)

New York JFK International Airport

The Oasis Day Spa is located at the JetBlue Airways Terminal 6. Treatments include Jet Set Facial Treatments at fifteen minutes for $30 and Frequent Flyer Back Treatments at thirty minutes for $60. (www.oasisdayspanyc.com)

The Molton Brown Travel Spa is located in the British Airways Lounge at Terminal 7. Treatments include Molton Brown Circulation Therapy and Molton Brown Shiatswe massages. The spa offers complimentary treatments to British Airways business and first-class passengers. (718-425-5849; www.moltonbrown.co.uk)

Newark Liberty International Airport

The Departure Spa has locations at both Terminal C at Gate 92 and Terminal B across from the duty-free shop. Treatments range from a Mini-Makeover ($30) to the Weary Traveler ($85), including a pedicure, a heated foot massage, and a nap. (http://departurespa.com)

The Massage Bar is located in Terminal A. A fifteen-minute seated massage runs $21; for thirty minutes it's $39. Another kiosk is located at the A3 connector. The Massage Bar also has locations at Washington-Dulles B Concourse, Nashville International B Concourse and C Concourse, and Seattle-Tacoma C Concourse and North Satellite. (http://massagebar.com)

San Francisco International Airport

XpresSpa, located in Gateway A, offers a variety of spa services such as the XpresSpa Stress & Tension Eliminator massage (twenty-five minutes for $45) and the XpresSpa Seaweed Facial (thirty minutes for $60). XpresSpa has additional locations at

JFK Terminals 1 and 4, as well as Pittsburgh International Terminals A and B. (www.xpresspa.com)

Vancouver International Airport

Vancouver International has three different spas (two partial-service kiosks in the airport proper and a full-service spa in the Fairmont Hotel Vancouver Airport). These spas offer everything from basic manicures and massages to specialized Y-Spas oriented toward men, which promise "nothing feminine" about services such as back waxing ($60) and sport massages ($115 for an hour). In addition, the airport-adjacent Fairmont Vancouver has a complete fitness center, where $15 gets you a full day of access to the health club, sauna, shower, and pool, and includes a locker for your luggage. (Fairmont Hotel Vancouver, 604-207-5200; www.absolutespa.com)

MORE FUN AT AIRPORTS

At many international airports, a long layover can actually be a refreshing and enjoyable experience.

Amsterdam

If Amsterdam's playful Schiphol Airport can't make you smile through your layover, you're a hardened traveler indeed. After all, what could be more fun than giant, people-shaped chairs and whimsical modern art?

But Schiphol's also packed with amenities. Feeling stiff after a long plane ride? Try a ten-minute "Back to Life" chair massage for €15 (about $18). If you're feeling intellectually depleted by the awful romantic comedies you sat through on the plane, head to the free Rijksmuseum beyond Passport Control between Piers E and F. There you'll find a rotation of temporary exhibitions alongside ten permanent works by Dutch Golden Age masters. And if that's not enough intellectual stimulation, check out two Dutch painters as they meticulously re-create Rembrandt's masterpiece, *Night Watch*. However, the new *Night Watch* will not be an exact copy, but instead will depict the scene a few moments later in time, with the same people in different poses.

Of course, if you're up for a taste of Amsterdam's vices, there's Holland Casino between Gates E and F, and available to any travelers age eighteen and over. You might lose weight by gambling—after all, it could be loosely classified as an exercise—but you're almost surely guaranteed to lose money. You can also eat well at Schiphol, which has its own supermarket, open from 6 A.M. until midnight. (www.schiphol.nl)

Auckland

If you get stuck Down Under, hope that your layover is in Auckland. It may seem staid compared with the overstimulation at Amsterdam's Schiphol or Singapore's Changi, but there's a lot to be said for an airport that's so resolutely pleasant. And like the rest of New Zealand, Auckland International offers a lot in the way of natural beauty and outdoor activities. For example, though Auckland doesn't have a gym in its terminals, the Flying Fit Health Club is located on airport land. To get there, stroll up Ray Emery Drive and take a right on Tom Pearce Drive. Keep walking past the roundabout to reach the club. It's a fifteen-minute walk so pleasant that most people skip public transit just to enjoy the fresh air.

Near the health club is the Aviation Country Club, featuring an eighteen-hole golf course. If you don't have the time, patience, or swing to play a full game of golf, there's also a mini–golf course, plus a driving range. Also in the works are several development projects that will add miles of walking trails in parklike areas near the airport that, while aimed at locals, will also be easily accessible to tourists. (www.auckland-airport.co.nz)

Johannesburg

Johannesburg, a major South African city for mining and industry, hasn't traditionally been known as a tourist destination. But
the city has begun to take advantage of the beauty of its natural
surroundings, offering tourists a number of relatively short and
reasonably inexpensive excursions. For 690 South African rand
(just over US$100), Siyabona Africa tours (www.siyabona.com)
offers its Night Game Drive & Cave Experience. This five-hour
tour with an English-speaking guide includes a nighttime jaunt
through a game reserve with lions, rhinos, and buffalo in an
open-air 4×4 vehicle. Then it's on to the Wonder Caves, with a
visit to the Cradle of Life—a look back at life 3.5 million years
ago. For 710 rand (about US$107), travelers can escape to the
Lesedi Cultural Village to experience a few hours of the natural
rhythms of African dance around a campfire with members of
the Zulu tribe.

Reykjavik

If you're on a layover in Reykjavik's Keflavik Airport, you're
probably flying on Icelandair, which offers some great deals on
transatlantic flights. Take advantage of these deals and love your
layover in Iceland. Get a natural high by turning a layover at Keflavik International into an hour-long soak in the Blue Lagoon,
one of Iceland's famed geothermal hot springs. It's just twenty
minutes from the terminal to the springs, which your body will
tell you are a natural wonder of the world. With Reykjavik Excursions (www.re.is), a nice soak is just $58, including round-
trip transportation from Keflavik.

Singapore

Asian airports are embracing their natural side. Kuala Lumpur
International features a rain forest arboretum and a playground
for kids. But it's Singapore's Changi International that really
fosters environmental appreciation (which is somewhat ironic

considering how technologically developed Singapore is today). There is a wide range of gardens scattered around the airport—including favorites like the rooftop Cactus Garden, the Sunflower Garden (with a maze!), and the Orchid Garden. And if you're unacquainted with the only fish that might be described as "regal," don't miss the koi ponds.

Of course, if you're craving more artificial fun, there's the giant 100-inch screen playing movies twenty-four hours a day in Terminal 2. And while many airports now offer massages, Singapore also boasts traditional Asian foot reflexology sessions. And what visit to Asia would be complete without a little karaoke? Not yours. Check out East & West Music Bar in Terminal 1 for a foot-stompin' good time. (www.changi.airport.com.sg)

GRAB A NAP

Between long layovers and delayed flights, sleeping in airports might seem like not just a good idea but a necessary one. However, before you try it, there are some things you need to know.

If you're looking for a quick nap, the transit lounges in most airports can do in a pinch. Of course, transit lounges aren't available in every airport—or to every traveler. But some airports, like those in Vancouver, Dubai, and Istanbul, do offer sleeping pods or by-the-hour airport hotels for naps. If you're stranded overnight in an airport due to flight delays, make sure to ask your airline for a hotel or sleeping pod voucher. At the very least, you should obtain access to the lounge facilities.

If a hotel or sleeping pod isn't available, and you're thinking about saving money by crashing at the airport, visit Sleeping InAirports.net. This site offers the inside scoop from other travelers on the best places to sleep at airports—and hands out the Golden Pillow award to the most sleep-friendly airports around the world. Singapore's Changi International has swept this category for several years, but a number of other airports, including those in Amsterdam, Auckland, Helsinki, Hong Kong, and Kuala Lumpur as well as Seoul's Incheon International have also made the list. They also issue the less-prestigious Poopy Airport Award to airports whose facilities fail to meet basic standards of safety, cleanliness, and comfort. Poopy Airport Awards were most recently handed out to Boston's Logan, Chicago's O'Hare, Paris's Charles de Gaulle, Moscow's Sheremetyevo, the airports in Cairo and Jakarta, and nearly all of the major airports in India.

When planning an overnight stay in an airport, or at least preparing for the possibility of one, it's important to bring the right gear. If you're a light sleeper, you'll definitely need a sleeping mask and earplugs. Headphones that cover your ears will help block out loud announcements. Bottled water and snacks are crucial for overnight stays, as most airport concessionaires will close at some point. Dressing in layers is helpful, since airport temperatures can range from subfreezing to sweltering. For airports that are less than clean, carrying sanitizing wipes is a good idea. And even if the airport is a Golden Pillow winner, packing books, cards, games, or music will prevent you from getting bored while you wait. Bring comfortable bedding, if possible, but be careful: Sleeping bags can attract the attention of airport security and lead to your unceremonious ejection from the airport. In fact, it's usually a good idea to be as friendly with the security staff as possible, especially in less-corrupt countries, where they won't demand a bribe. In some airports, not only will security help you find a good place to sleep, but they'll help keep an eye on your bags.

Once you're bedded down for the evening, there are some other important things to keep in mind. No matter how much of an airport pro you are, don't act like it. Remember, an airport isn't a hotel—a sob story about being forced to spend the night there will get you further than an attitude of entitlement. If you're worried your alarm clock might not wake you, or you don't have an alarm clock, some intrepid travelers have even been known to place a few Post-it Notes saying "Please Wake Me at 6:00 A.M." on their person. This can actually do the trick. And finally, it's important to always have a backup plan. Not all airport officials think airport sleeping should be allowed. So if you're sleeping in an airport, be prepared to explain why you're there and show proof that you do have a flight the next day.

LONG LAYOVERS ARE YOUR FRIEND: FINDING A GYM

The best thing to do when you are stuck between flights, or when your flight is delayed, is . . . exercise. Some airports have gyms inside, like these:

- Chicago O'Hare
  Hilton Hotel
  Located in terminal
  www.hilton.com
  773-601-1723

The O'Hare Hilton has a full-service fitness center with various types of machines and free weights available. There's also a swimming pool, Jacuzzi, steam room, and sauna accessible to those who've purchased a day pass to the fitness facilities. For additional fees, they also offer basic spa services such as massages and tanning beds. Passes start at $10 per day. Naturally, Hilton guests may access these facilities for free.

- Las Vegas McCarran International
  24-Hour Fitness
  Located in terminal
  www.ncjournalforwomen.com
  702-261-3971

- Miami International
  Miami International Airport Hotel
  Located in terminal
  http://miami.citysearch.com
  800-327-1276

- Vancouver International
  Spa at the Fairmont Hotel
  Located in terminal
  www.yvr.ca
  604-248-2772

But if you're not lucky enough to be in an airport that has a gym, most airports do have gyms nearby.

Atlanta Hartsfield-Jackson

Although some hotels near Atlanta's Hartsfield-Jackson International Airport claim to offer fitness centers, most are little more than one room with a few pieces of equipment. Travelers interested in a more serious workout head to Holland Fitness, twenty or thirty minutes by taxi from Hartsfield-Jackson International. Offering day passes for just $8, Holland Fitness boasts a host of classes, the latest equipment, showers, lockers, and even child care. Take a basic aerobics course or kick and punch away stress with kickboxing and karate classes. Chiropractic care, massages, and tanning beds are among the extra goodies that the club offers. Holland Fitness is open Monday through Thursday from 5 A.M. to 7 P.M., Friday from 5 A.M. to 10 P.M., Saturday from 7 A.M. to 10 P.M., and Sunday from 10 A.M. to 6 P.M. (770-222-9116; www.hollandfitness.com)

Dallas–Fort Worth International

Dallas–Fort Worth International has several exercise facilities on-site, but unfortunately, most are not available to the average traveler. For example, there's a little-known workout room in the American Airlines Admirals Club. I discovered it totally by accident one day, and ended up on the elliptical for thirty minutes between flights. One caution: If you're not a member, it will cost you a rather expensive $50 for a day pass—almost the price of a local hotel room—but that will get you access to the workout facilities as well as the Internet and the quiet lounge facilities.

While there is a spa, pool, and exercise room at the Grand Hyatt in Terminal 1, you must be a guest to use the equipment. Fortunately, the Irving Fitness airport location is just ten minutes by taxi from the terminals. Irving Fitness offers day passes for a steep $20 a day, but weekly passes are only $25. Guests at the airport-adjacent Clarion Inn get free access, and a number of local hotels also offer $10-a-day discounts. The day pass includes access to step, PiYo, and Pilates classes. Irving Fitness offers the normal complement of cardio and weight machines, but no pool, Jacuzzi, or steam room. However, a great advantage of Irving Fitness is that it's open twenty-four hours a day during the week, with long hours on the weekends as well. Irving Fitness Airport is located at 3909 West Airport Freeway, Suite 200, in Irving. (972-257 0221)

A cheaper option to get in a day's workout in the Dallas–Fort Worth area is the Bally Total Fitness location at 2715 North Belt Line Road in Irving, just over 4 miles from the terminals. While not all Bally members can visit gyms nationwide (this option is available only on certain plans), the day-pass rate for nonmembers is just $10. This club is highly recommended for avid swimmers, offering a heated pool, hot tub, and saunas in the men's and women's locker rooms. This location also offers a number of group exercise classes and a more-than-adequate selection of equipment. Open Monday through Thursday 5 A.M. to 11 P.M., Friday 5 A.M. to 10 P.M., and Saturday and Sunday 8 A.M. to 7 P.M. (972-252-8772; www.ballyfitness.com)

Detroit Metropolitan Wayne County

While there are no workout facilities available on-site at Detroit's Metro Wayne County International, plenty of exercise options are available nearby. The Westin Detroit Metropolitan Airport Hotel, less than a mile from the terminals, does have a workout room for its guests and those willing to pay for a day pass ($10). The best thing about the Westin Detroit's facilities is that they're open twenty-four hours a day, so you can exercise even on a late-night layover. Arrangements for the use of this facility must be obtained through the hotel. (734-942-6500; www.starwoodhotels.com/westin)

A bit farther away is the Wayne Racquet & Exercise Club at 4635 Howe Road, about fifteen minutes by taxi from the terminals. For just $7, travelers can take advantage of a number of different amenities. In addition to the weight room, cardio room, and the courts you'd expect from a racquet club, there's a large pool, wet and dry sauna, whirlpool, waterslides, an indoor track, and women-specific facilities. The Wayne Racquet & Exercise Club is open Monday through Friday 6 A.M. to 9 P.M., Saturday 8 A.M. to 9 P.M., and Sunday 9 A.M. to 9 P.M. (734-728-2900)

Houston Bush Intercontinental

About ten or fifteen minutes by taxi from Houston's Bush Intercontinental Airport is 24-Hour Fitness. Living up to its name, this location is open twenty-four hours a day for travelers who might not be accustomed to the time zone in Texas. 24-Hour Fitness offers day passes for $15 for those who don't have memberships. In addition to aquatic facilities such as the pool, sauna, and steam room, this location offers a wide variety of classes—everything from cardio and step to hip-hop and Pilates. Most are offered from 5:30 to 11:00 A.M. and from 5 to 8 P.M. (281-812-3059; www.24hourfitness.com)

Phoenix Sky Harbor

In Phoenix, about five miles from Sky Harbor Airport, there's a top-notch LA Fitness club. Exercise addicts can choose from offerings of more than eighty classes per week, including yoga, cycling, Pilates, cardio kickboxing, club boxing, and various aerobics disciplines. The facility also boasts all brand-new equipment. A day pass is $15, but elite membership gives nationwide access to all LA Fitness locations for $49 a month with a $149 registration fee. (602-241-9800; www.lafitness.com)

Salt Lake City International

Salt Lake City's gym scene is notable for a great reason: low prices. Here, travelers should skip the gym chains and seek out some independent options that are both closer to the airport and significantly cheaper for a day pass.

Most clubs that offer day passes for just $4.50 are marked by a distinct lack of clean, modern facilities and amenities. Not so with Magna Fitness & Recreation, located just ten to fifteen minutes by taxi from the terminals. Here you'll find all the necessary equipment for a complete workout, plus an indoor track, basketball courts, and an outdoor pool. Magna Gym is open Monday through Thursday 5 A.M. to 10 P.M., Friday 5 A.M. to 9 P.M., Saturday 7 A.M. to 7 P.M., and Sunday 10 A.M. to 3 P.M. and is located at 8400 West, 3270 South in Magna. (801-250-2194)

Alternatively, there's the Salt Lake City Sports Complex, just fifteen minutes by taxi from the terminals. This is an especially good choice for families, thanks to its myriad kid-friendly activities such as ice skating. The SLC Sports Complex features a full array of workout equipment; classes including spin, Pilates, and yoga; all kinds of sports; and the massive Steiner Aquatic Center. For access to all of this, you'll pay just $6 for a day pass. The SLC Sports Complex is located at 645 South Guardsmen Way (580 East) in Salt Lake City and is open Monday through Friday 5 A.M. to 10 P.M., Saturday 6 A.M. to

9 P.M., and Sunday 10 A.M. to 4 P.M. (801-583-9713; www
.sportscomplex.slco.org)

San Francisco International

There are a number of great exercise options for travelers near San
Francisco International Airport (SFO). Both nearby YMCA
locations—in Stonestown (twenty or twenty-five minutes by taxi)
and Peninsula (fifteen minutes by taxi)—offer extensive workout
facilities, plus lap pools and basketball and volleyball courts for
$10 to $12 per day pass. (www.ymca.com)

The Touchstone Climbing & Fitness Centers in Mission
Cliffs, about fifteen minutes by taxi from the airport, will really
make an SFO layover a fun experience. Mission Cliffs has
14,000 square feet of climbable terrain, walls over 50 feet high,
dry saunas, an extensive weight room, and a warehouse-type
atmosphere. Equipment rentals are available for those travelers
who might have forgotten to pack their rock-climbing shoes.
Day passes run just $8 to $16, depending on the facilities you
want to use, and the center is open Monday through Friday from
6:30 A.M. to 10 P.M. and Saturday and Sunday from 10 A.M. to
6 P.M. (415-550-0515)

Washington, D.C., Dulles International

While Washington's Dulles International Airport doesn't have
an exercise facility on-site, there are a number of good clubs just
a short taxi ride away. A Gold's Gym is available in Chantilly,
Virginia, just under 4 miles from the airport. But in Washington
D.C., it's the independent gyms that represent the best nearby
workout options.

Olympus Gym is closest to Dulles, at about 2.6 miles. For
$10, travelers have access to all of the basic workout facilities—
cardio equipment and weight machines, free weights, and cable
machines. It's a low/no-frills place, but it's great for a quick
workout. Located at 308 Glenn Drive in Sterling, Virginia,

Olympus Gym is open Monday through Friday 5 A.M. to 11 P.M. and Saturday and Sunday 8 A.M. to 8 P.M. (703-430-0666)

Travelers who have a little more time and an interest in some serious physical fitness should head to the Worldgate Club, a fifteen-minute taxi ride from Dulles. While day passes are a steep $25, you'll get free access if you're staying at the airport Marriott. Of course, $25 isn't unreasonable, given the number of amenities and exercise options at the club. The Worldgate Club offers a pool—the only nearby club to do so—in its three-story facility topped by a skylight. There are racquetball, squash, and basketball courts; a wide array of new equipment; and a huge, ever-evolving variety of classes—including six types of yoga, cardio kickboxing, step aerobics, Zumba, and many types of dance. Open 5 A.M. to 11 P.M. Monday through Friday and 7 A.M. to 8 P.M. weekends, World Gate Club is as good as it gets at Dulles. (703-709-9100)

Some honorable mentions and surprises:

There's a partly wooded 12-mile biking and hiking trail that circles Baltimore-Washington International airport. And in Germany, bring your bathing suit—the Munich airport features a lap pool at the Kempinski airport hotel (for $18, you get lockers and towels).

WALK IT OFF

If you don't have time to escape from the airport for a workout, there's always the option of walking the terminals themselves.

Atlanta Hartsfield-Jackson International

An underground corridor, which links all terminals, is 1.25 miles one way, making a complete loop of $2^1/_2$ miles. Pick up the underground corridor instead of taking the train from the main terminal and proceed to the end of it.

Boston Logan International

Here are some possibilities for your walking course:

Terminal A main building	1,377 feet
Terminal A walkway to satellite building	876 feet
Terminal A Satellite Terminal	997 feet
Terminal B American Airlines side	1,814 feet
Terminal B US Airways side	1,267 feet
Terminal C	1,982 feet
Terminal D	816 feet
Terminal E	2,897 feet

Chicago O'Hare

The best walking exercise to be had at O'Hare is in the biggest terminal, Terminal 3. A steady walk to the end of each of the four concourses and back takes approximately thirty-five minutes and is, very roughly, a mile. And outside the security boundary, you can walk the entire three-terminal length, which runs $1\frac{1}{2}$ miles, or 3 miles round-trip.

Cincinnati–Northern Kentucky International

It's not a fun walk, but you'll get your exercise going from the main Delta terminal to the Comair flights.

Dallas–Fort Worth International

The airport is very proud of its new skylink train, which is a tremendous improvement over the old automated tram. But if you're not outrageously late for your connecting flight, you can easily get in about $2\frac{1}{2}$ miles of walking from Gate C11-12, up through Terminal D, connecting to Terminal B, around the half-mile oval, over the sky bridge, through four terminals out of five. (www.dfwairport.com)

Denver International

In Denver, you must take trams between terminals. The distances inside each terminal (from one end to the other, not round-trip) are as follows:

Concourse A	1,832 feet
Concourse B	3,300 feet
Concourse C	1,512 feet

Detroit Metro Wayne County

It's actually possible to walk a 3-mile loop inside the terminals at this airport. Simply start at either end of Terminal A (avoid the moving walkways for maximum effect, obviously) and walk the length to the tunnel to Terminal B, continue to that terminal's end, loop around, and return to the beginning of Terminal A. All told, that's nearly 3 miles, without the need for additional security checks. For a 1-mile walk, try ambling the length of just Terminal A. (www.metroairport.com)

Houston Bush Intercontinental

There's an interterminal train running the length of the airport, and the carpeted area alongside it is a popular place to run or walk. It's 5,036 feet from one end of the train loop to the other. It's always cool down there; unobstructed it's a 2-mile round-trip.

Kansas City International

Each of the three terminals is connected by shuttle bus, and walking between them really isn't an option. Essentially, each gate has its own security, so there's no walking once you are inside the security perimeter. However, you can walk around the terminal, on the inside or the outside, for half a mile. A complete loop from one end to the other and back again would be right around 1 mile.

Las Vegas McCarran

All distances measured are beyond the security checkpoints and include one round-trip walk of each gate area from the security checkpoint to the farthest point. All distances are approximate.

Beyond A/B Security Checkpoint
   A Gates: .5 mile
   B Gates: .5 mile
   A and B Gates combined: 1 mile
Beyond C/D Security Checkpoint
   C Gates: .70 mile
   D Gates: .92 mile
   (It is not possible to walk between the C and D gates.)

Los Angeles International

Each terminal has different security checkpoints, and it's not possible to move between them (except that you can walk inside the security area between Terminals 6 and 7). These are the distances from security to the end of the terminal, one way.

Terminal 1	Approximately 525 feet
Terminal 2	Approximately 432 feet
Terminal 3	Approximately 544 feet
Terminal 4	Approximately 727 feet
Terminal 5	Approximately 665 feet
Terminal 6	Approximately 867 feet
Terminal 7	Approximately 672 feet
Terminal 8	Approximately 797 feet
Tom Bradley International Terminal	Approximately 1,008 feet (for each wing)

Miami International

This airport is U-shaped. Officially, you can't go from concourse to concourse as a ticketed passenger inside security. But you actually *can* go from Concourse E to D to C, and the total distance is more than a mile. If you want to walk outside of security, consider these numbers: From one end of the terminal to the other 2,500 feet. It's the same distance on the upper and the lower level.

Minneapolis–St. Paul International

After you've entered the security area, one course around the main terminal (Lindbergh) is a 1½-mile loop that includes lots of window-shopping and is the recommended walk for this airport. The smaller Humphrey Terminal is just ¼ mile across. (612-726-5555; www.mspairport.com)

New York JFK

JFK's eight operating terminals are located in a circle around the central terminal area. The distances between terminals that are given here are approximate. However, you should not assume that a short distance indicates that you should plan to walk between terminals. The best and safest way for getting between terminals is the AirTrain. It is easy and convenient. However, if you want to walk between *certain* terminals at JFK, here are some distances:

Terminal 2 (300 feet across) and Terminal 3 are connected by an enclosed, elevated pedestrian walkway that is 700 feet long.

Terminal 8 and Terminal 9 are connected by an interior concourse and a ground-level sidewalk (each is 700 feet across with 200 feet of sidewalk).

Terminal 4, main terminal, B Concourse, from Gate 20 to the end, is 1,314 feet, 6 inches, and from the back line of the headhouse (main building) it is 1,147 feet.

Terminal 4, main terminal, A Concourse is 673 feet, 6 inches.

The total width of the headhouse is 960 feet.

New York LaGuardia

All distances are for areas outside security along front sidewalks.

Length of Delta terminal	550 feet
Between Delta and US Airways terminals	300 feet
Length of US Airways Terminal	1,100 feet
From US Airways Terminal to Main Terminal	1,200 feet
Length of Main Terminal half-loop	1,350 feet

Inside security:

Concourse A	250 feet
Concourse B	350 feet
Concourse C	400 feet
Concourse D	500 feet

It's not possible to move between concourses without going through security again.

Newark Liberty International

These distances are postsecurity inside the airport:

Terminal A	850 feet
From Terminal A to Terminal B	1,100 feet
Terminal B	850 feet
From Terminal B to Terminal C	1,100 feet
Terminal C	850 feet
Total (beginning of A to end of C)	4,750 feet, almost a mile

Orlando International

If you walk the main terminal, presecurity, one complete lap around the rectangle totals 2,090 feet. Terminals themselves are too small for good walking—they are less than 500 feet. There are no workout facilities on-site—not even in the lounges.

Phoenix Sky Harbor International

In Terminal 4, with 75 percent of the passenger traffic, you can loop around between the concourses in (almost) a square. Each

Terminal 4 concourse varies in length; the ones on the north side are 600 feet long, and the ones on the south side are 300 to 330 feet long. The squared loop between the concourses (inside secure Terminal 4) is the longest walkway—currently it's in a horseshoe shape, and the longest one-way walk is 5,300 feet. (It will eventually be expanded to complete a square.)

Terminal 3   700 feet length of concourse
Terminal 2   800 feet length of concourse

Other terminals have much less walking capacity—just the length of the individual concourse, as indicated.

Salt Lake City International

Within the two terminals, there's a system of five concourses of differing lengths with a connector linking each, and enterprising travelers can power-walk these concourses. The distance of each concourse is measured from end-to-end, not round-trip.

Connector length   2,281 feet
Concourse lengths:
  A   493 feet
  B   1,089 feet
  C   671 feet
  D   665 feet
  E   366 feet

The airport-adjacent three-level parking structure is also good for walking (employees use it for exercise). (www.slcairport.com)

San Francisco International

A full circle just inside the airport is 1 mile for nonticketed passengers. The maximum walk is 1/2 mile for ticketed passengers inside security.

Washington, D.C., Dulles International

Starting at Gate A1 and walking to Gate B52, round-trip, is just over a mile. A round-trip between Terminals C and D is approximately 1.5 miles. (www.mwaa.com)

Gate A1 to Gate B52 (inside security)	2,936 feet
Concourse A	1,010 feet
B	1,926 feet
C and D, end-to-end	3,917 feet

Washington, D.C., Ronald Reagan

Walking to the end of Terminal A–C, presecurity, is .65 mile one way. Once inside, there's not much room to really get your stroll on.

There's no doubt that you can benefit from walking. But no amount of walking can properly prepare you for your next challenge: sitting, endlessly, on airplanes . . .

CHAPTER 4

On the Plane

You've run the gauntlet through the airport. And you got through it without succumbing to Mr. Goodbar, or even that oversauced turkey wrap. Now you've finally reached your gate, and with any luck, in a few minutes, you'll be on the plane and in your seat.

But once you board, you discover that you have no room, and the guy sitting beside you has spread out his supersized Coke and McDonald's burger right next to you. Boy, those fries smell good!

You resist the fries, but you can't ignore . . . the size.

No matter how you situate yourself, you find your flesh in contact with his. Is it your imagination, or are airline seats getting smaller? Sorry, folks, but as small as the seats seem, as uncomfortable as it is to have your knees wrapped around your neck in coach, the truth is that the seats aren't smaller—you've gotten *bigger*. I'm sad to report that the plane isn't the only widebody rolling down the runway.

If you ever needed more incentive to lose weight on the road, keep reading.

In 1995, the Federal Aviation Administration set the recommended average weight per adult passenger, which is used to calculate aircraft loads, at 180 pounds in the summer and 185 pounds in the winter. That's heavy enough, right? Not exactly. After the deadly crash of a commuter plane in Charlotte, North Carolina, in January 2003, investigators determined that the weight of those on board might actually have been a factor in the tragedy. As a result, the FAA ordered airlines to add 10 pounds to the assumed average weight of each passenger when calculating aircraft loads.

And that's just the beginning.

In 2005, the Centers for Disease Control measured the economic and environmental costs of obesity on airlines. As the mean weight of an American adult rose nearly 10 pounds during the 1990s, this extra weight translated into more fuel being spent by the airlines and more pollution in the environment. A lot more.

The CDC's study cites U.S. Department of Transportation estimates that it takes a gallon of jet fuel to transport 7.3 tons of passengers or cargo 1 mile by air, and air travelers flew approximately 515 billion passenger-miles in the United States in 2000. Given the extra 10 pounds per passenger, roughly an extra 350 million gallons of jet fuel were consumed to carry the additional weight. That translates to about $275 million to transport those extra pounds of fat. And for the environment, that's about 3.8 million tons of carbon dioxide emissions as well as smaller quantities of other pollutants.

How's that airborne Big Mac sound right about now?

I've said it before, but it bears repeating. Most airline food is unappealing. People don't eat it because they're hungry, they eat it because they're *bored*.

But the real questions are *what* are you eating—and how much? And what are you drinking? And, last but not least, *why*?

First, some history.

Since the first record of airline food being served—on July 30, 1927—people have seen a downward spiral in not only the quality of the food, but its nutritional content. And while the airline food industry is worth $20 billion a year worldwide and employs 100,000 people, you'd never guess that by observing what they serve you. To add insult to injury, both the way food tastes and our appetites for it change at flight altitudes.

Peter Jones, who is actually professor of airline food at the University of Surrey in England, has, as you might suspect, studied the subject. He reports that the flavors of foods become less distinct at such altitudes and the aroma of wine is diminished. At higher altitudes, many people react more strongly to caffeine. Furthermore, the low humidity in the plane's cabin (less than 25 percent) dries the mucous membranes lining the nasal cavity and reduces the sense of smell. Similarly, the dryness of the mouth affects the taste receptors. According to Jones, in-flight atmospheric pressure conditions in commercial jet aircraft (at 5,000 to 8,000 feet) are similar to what mountain climbers experience. It has been suggested that the lower cabin pressure and the associated moderate lack of oxygen causes, as Jones notes, a "sluggish effect on digestion and absorption of nutrients."

And here's another reason to avoid that Big Mac on the plane. Jones's research indicates that the aircraft cabin pressure also causes gases from fatty foods in the body to expand. "The physiological effects of traveling at altitude are analogous to those observed in climbers," he says, "and hence airlines should recognize and attempt to respond appropriately to maximize passenger satisfaction for example by:

- Providing opportunities for smaller meals more frequently on demand,

- Proactively addressing the water balance problem through passenger education and the availability of drinking water,

- Providing meals that are easy to digest and taste good."

Of course, none of the airlines I know do that.

This once again raises the question: Why are you eating on the plane?

TO EAT OR NOT TO EAT

As airlines cut back on food, many of them are now offering snack boxes in lieu of a real meal. Although you'd think a snack would be light on calories, you'd better look at what's inside.

When the Center for Science in the Public Interest actually counted up what was offered in a Southwest Snack Pack on a flight from Los Angeles to Nashville, here is what they found: six Golden Oreo cookies (250 calories), six Ritz Crackers with Real Cheese (200 calories), and a bag of fruit-flavored Jell-O Gelatin Snacks (90 calories). They point out that that little box contains more than 25 percent of a day's allotment of calories for white flour, fat, sugar, and salt. You might think the cheese and crackers would provide some protein, but you get only 2 grams—no more than in the six-packs of Oreos. They also point out that the Gelatin Snack is mostly sugar with a little grape and cherry juice mixed in for taste.

The point is that you should bring your own snacks. Or at least pick up some nuts in the airport before you board. A recent survey asked flight attendants if they eat the food they serve on their flights. More than a third responded, "Only if desperate." You don't have to be desperate. You just have to be smart.

Here's what my nutritionist, Heidi Skolnik, recommends:

- Unsalted nuts

- Raw veggies

- String cheese

- Dried fruit (personal favorites are apricots and almonds, cashews, and walnuts, but I don't mind hazelnuts and some peanuts thrown in!)

- Fresh fruit

- Granola bars

- Hard-boiled eggs

- Sports drinks

- Yogurt

- Dry cereal, such as a baggie of Cheerios

The athletes she works with will pack individual bags or small cans of tuna, small jars of peanut butter, whole grain crackers, energy bars, and dried soups in a cup (you can always get hot water even at convenience stores and on a plane).

If you are flying more than a few hours, however, it can be difficult to turn down the airline meal—that is, if it's served at all. On a recent American Airlines flight, I was offered the choice between a lethal cheese pizza and a somewhat less scary roast beef sandwich. I chose the sandwich. When the tray arrived, this is what was on it:

- A tiny salad

- A sandwich consisting of a thin slice of roast beef wedged between two huge pieces of bread

- Cookies, for dessert

I took apart the sandwich and ate just the meat—which, by the way, I was able to consume in one mouthful, it was *that* minuscule. The bread actually camouflaged how small the portion was. I ate the salad with minimal dressing, but then came the challenge: Dessert. A quick glance at the back of this package of walnut shortbread cookies revealed what I had feared: The three small cookies inside contained 140 calories, 8 grams of fat, 1.5 grams of saturated fat, 65 milligrams of sodium, 15 grams of carbs, and a whopping 1 gram of protein. I stared at that bag of cookies for the entire flight . . . and then I gave it to my seatmate. Hooray for me.

AIRLINE MEALS

Let's face it. The best thing about airline food is that the portions are small. And that is if you get served anything at all.

The numbers might surprise you, however. Even with airlines cutting back, there are still three billion meals served on planes every year.

And how much do the airlines spend—per passenger—on what they call food? During the first six months of the most recent reporting period, this is what the major carriers spent per passenger for domestic flights:

American	$3.88
Continental	$3.67
Delta	$2.87
Northwest	$1.95
United	$3.43

Compare that to the budget carriers:

America West	55¢
Southwest	23¢

In Europe, meals are still considered important—and they are expected on flights. British Airways' catering at Heathrow is most likely the largest single food outlet in the world, supplying eighty thousand meals per day—not just to BA flights, but to many different airlines that subcontract them to cook and deliver meals for their flights.

When you consider the sheer volume involved, it's amazing that more people don't get sick just from the food. Indeed, there have been problems in the past—which is another reason not to eat airline meals. Between August 2003 and August 2004, investigators in the United Kingdom found some meals that were infected with bacteria that cause food poisoning. Worse, they found *E. coli* in a lemon chicken salad and a prawn-with-lemon-herbs dish as well.

In fairness, however, the actual frequency of such incidents is so low as to be considered insignificant. The real issue is whether you need to eat on planes. We are, after all, creatures of habit—so much so that Pavlov and his dogs would be proud of us. And we've been conditioned to eat six miles up.

Want proof? I am convinced there are people out there who have no life and actually fly *because* the airline is serving a meal on board. These people are so obsessed with this that there is a website that allows you to see what's being served in the air before you get to the airport. If you must (and *only* if you must), go to www.airlinemeals.net, where people take pictures of what they're serving and post them for others to see and share. Not a pretty site.

One of the first things Heidi Skolnik told me is that airplane food is extremely high in both fat and calories—even the so-called light snacks. Even worse, in order to keep the food moist in the dehydrated airline environment, airline chefs tend to smother everything in thick mystery sauces. Until recently, airlines tended to serve high-fat food because not only is it cheaper and easy to reheat, but it also makes people tired (a great thing for harried flight attendants).

So, if they're still available, try the low-fat or vegetarian options. Or even skip the meal altogether if you have eaten before the flight or you know you will eat soon after arrival.

One more thing to remember: Because of the altitude, flying reduces the functioning of the taste buds by a third, so if you think airline food tastes bad in the air, just imagine what it would taste like on the ground! And although the portion size of American food is getting larger, airline food still has to fit in those little boxes on the tray.

One of the best meal options was sold on Song, Delta's now-defunct budget airline. For $8, you could get an organic meal planned by Peter Davis, from the organic restaurant Henrietta's Table at the Charles Hotel in Cambridge, Massachusetts. The meals were so popular that they almost always sold out and you had to preorder online to make sure your selection was available. A typical dish, Grilled Chicken Niçoise Salad, consisted of a bed of Earthbound Farm organic romaine lettuce topped with grilled breast of herbed chicken strips, blanched green beans, kalamata olives, ripe cherry tomatoes, and new potatoes, all drizzled with balsamic vinaigrette dressing. I'd be happy to pay the $8 for *that* in-flight offering. Another option was the BBQ Chicken and Black Bean Salad: grilled barbecue-rubbed chicken breast with black bean, red pepper, and corn chili served on a bed of Earthbound Farm organic romaine lettuce, with a side of red pepper vinaigrette dressing, also for $8. Hungry yet?

But since you don't get to eat that now, you are once again faced with the usual poor choices. So how do you select your meal? Though we contacted all the major airlines, none of them would volunteer any helpful information about the meals they serve. Even Sky Chefs, one of the large airline caterers, wouldn't cooperate. "We look at our food as restaurant food," said spokesperson Roxanne Conrad. "Nutritional information is not available."

Actually, it *is* available. I just had to ask someone else to find it for me.

AIRLINE-BY-AIRLINE ANALYSIS

Enter the Physicians Committee for Responsible Medicine, a nonprofit group of doctors based in Washington, D.C. Their nutritionists reviewed menus from eighteen airlines to determine the healthfulness of their in-flight meals. Healthy items were presumed to be high in fiber and low in fat, saturated fat, and cholesterol. Their investigators collected hundreds of airline menus, then used a nutritional software program to analyze the food offerings to help you make better choices. The chart on pages 118 to 127 presents their results. Though the numbers are approximate, they do give you a very helpful ballpark figure of what's really in that anonymous chicken sandwich.

Domestic Airlines

America West
America West offers first-class passengers a very limited choice of healthy alternatives, such as a vegetarian breakfast of fresh fruit and granola. First-class passengers can also make advance requests for healthier fare, including couscous with apricots, apricot and raisin compote, and broiled tomato at breakfast and a portobello mushroom sandwich and fresh fruit at lunch or dinner. But coach passengers are not given these options; they are limited to purchasing meals and snacks from the In-Flight Café, which offers the high-fat Egg, Peppered Turkey, and Swiss Toaster and other unhealthful options.

Meal service overview: Serves complimentary meals to customers in first class on domestic flights longer than three hours that depart between 6 A.M. and 7:30 P.M. Pure vegetarian/vegan special meals are an option only in first class and on certain flights. Other travelers can buy meals from the In-Flight Café.

American Airlines
Main Cabin Snack Service has replaced most complimentary meals on coach domestic flights. Unfortunately, all these choices are less than healthy. The snack boxes contain prepackaged items such as cheese, crackers, sausage, and cookies. When sandwiches and wraps are offered, they are filled with fatty and cholesterol-laden ingredients, such as the Ham and Cheddar Twister Club Sandwich, which contains ham, cheddar cheese, bacon strips, and mayonnaise.

PCRM's Nutritional Analysis of Airline Menu Items

Airline	Menu item	Calories	Milligrams of cholesterol	Grams of fat	Percentage of calories from fat	Grams of saturated fat	Percentage of calories from saturated fat
America West	Couscous with apricots, apricot and raisin compote, and broiled tomato (*special meal, first class, domestic*)	213	0	1	4%	<1	1%
	Turkey, ham, and Swiss with cream cheese on a nine-grain roll, with fresh fruit (*first class, domestic*)						
	Egg, Peppered Turkey, and Swiss Toaster — thinly sliced peppered turkey, scrambled eggs, and Swiss cheese between two slices of cinnamon swirl French toast, with dijonnaise	448	80	20	41%	11	23%

	504	405	27	47%	9	16%
American on the side (buy-on-board, coach, domestic)						
Orzo antipasto salad, roll, margarine, fruit dessert (special meal, first or business class, domestic)	367	0	12	29%	2	5%
Ham and Cheddar Twister Club Sandwich—smoked ham, green leaf lettuce, tomatoes, cheddar cheese, and bacon strips on a Danish roll, with a side of mayonnaise spread (buy-on-board, coach, domestic)	466	72	28	54%	10	19%
Rosemary-roasted double lamb chops, merlot sauce, broccoli-tomato medley, yellow potato wedges with thyme (first class)	960	211	65	61%	28	26%

PCRM's Nutritional Analysis of Airline Menu Items (*Continued*)

Airline	Menu item	Calories	Milligrams of cholesterol	Grams of fat	Percentage of calories from fat	Grams of saturated fat	Percentage of calories from saturated fat
Continental	Grilled tenderloin of beef with creamy herb sauce, with twice-baked potato with bacon (*business, first, international*)	951	104	53	50%	14	13%
	Personal cheese pizza (*coach, domestic*)	812	25	27	30%	12	13%
	Beef charbroil burger (*coach, domestic*)	320	50	16	45%	6	17%
Delta	Cheese omelet, turkey Canadian bacon, roasted potatoes, blueberry muffin, and fresh fruit (*coach, domestic*)	616	576	30	44%	13	19%
	Turkey and Swiss cheese sandwich, potato chips, cookie (*coach, domestic*)	486	47	22	41%	7	13%

	Duck breast with barbecue sauce, herb and cheese grits, zucchini, corn and tomato medley (business class, international)	390	67	15%	1	3%
	Chicken Caesar salad, with breadsticks and fresh fruit (business class, international)	624	70	23%	4	6%
Northwest	Vegetarian wrap (buy-on-board, domestic)	167	0	19%	1	4%
	Deli meat sandwich (buy-on-board, domestic)	232	31	21%	1	5%
United	Seasonal fruit platter with cereal (first and business class)	203	0	10%	<1	2%
	Tomato and chive omelet with hollandaise sauce and fresh seasonal fruit, with asiago potato pie, sautéed pork sausage, and Black Forest ham (first and business class)	700	493	63%	17	22%

PCRM's Nutritional Analysis of Airline Menu Items (*Continued*)

Airline	Menu item	Calories	Milligrams of cholesterol	Grams of fat	Percentage of calories from fat	Grams of saturated fat	Percentage of calories from saturated fat
United	Tuscan Wrap—marinated roasted chicken breast, Genoa salami, provolone cheese, roasted red tomatoes, kalamata olives, basil and garlic cream cheese, in low-carb tortilla wrap (*buy-on-board, coach, domestic*)	461	93	30	59%	14	28%
	Turkey Cobb Salad—turkey breast, sliced tomato, Swiss cheese, olives, sliced eggs, bacon, romaine lettuce, and ranch dressing, with fresh seasonal mixed fruit (*buy-on-board, coach, domestic*)	560	170	35	56%	11	17%

Air New Zealand	New Zealand lamb with horopito salt, carrot puree, and snow peas (business class)	208	97	7	32%	3	13%
British Airways	Spicy warm vegetable salad (first class)	25	0	<1	6%	<1	1%
	Fresh salad leaves with balsamic vinaigrette (first class)	37	1	3	77%	<1	6%
	Penne pasta with tomato and olive ragout (first class)	309	0	7	19%	1	3%
	Fresh seasonal fruit plate (first class)	92	0	1	5%	<1	1%
	Tempeh cakes with sweet chili dipping sauce (first class)	285	0	15	47%	3	10%
	Fresh salad leaves with tomato and basil oil (first class)	37	1	3	77%	<1	6%
	Grilled fillet steak with port wine sauce, chanterelle mushrooms, Vichy carrots, broccolini, and olive oil mashed potatoes (first class)	493	68	26	47%	8	15%

PCRM's Nutritional Analysis of Airline Menu Items *(Continued)*

Airline	Menu item	Calories	Milligrams of cholesterol	Grams of fat	Percentage of calories from fat	Grams of saturated fat	Percentage of calories from saturated fat
British Airways	Full English breakfast—scrambled eggs, bacon, pork sausages, sautéed mushrooms, grilled tomatoes, hash brown potatoes (*first class*)	906	511	70	70%	26	25%
Cathay Pacific	Penne pasta primavera (*coach, international*)	343	0	5	13%	1	2%
	Omelet with grilled bacon, croquette potatoes, sautéed mushroom and tomato stew (*economy, international*)	536	586	34	57%	9	16%
	Grilled New York steak with shallot demiglaze, stuffed baked potatoes, buttered green beans, and carrots (*first class, international*)	716	84	18	23%	7	9%

Airline	Menu item						
	...scallion oyster sauce, egg fried rice, and sautéed vegetables (*business class, international*)	278	100	9	30%	2	7%
Japan Airlines	Tandoori chicken, marinated shrimp, soft salami, and curry-flavor potato salad (*coach, international*)	587	355	32	50%	9	14%
	Grilled beef fillet with Café de Paris butter, Anna potatoes, and zucchini and carrots (*business class, international*)	476	84	26	49%	11	21%
	Waldorf salad (*business class, international*)	271	14	23	75%	3	10%
	Barley red pepper corn salad with lettuce leaf liner (*coach, international*)	169	0	4	19%	<1	1%
Lufthansa	Grilled vegetables— portobello mushroom, Japanese eggplant, squash, tomatoes, and asparagus (*business class, international*)	128	0	1	7%	<1	2%

PCRM's Nutritional Analysis of Airline Menu Items *(Continued)*

Airline	Menu item	Calories	Milligrams of cholesterol	Grams of fat	Percentage of calories from fat	Grams of saturated fat	Percentage of calories from saturated fat
Lufthansa	Marinated mushrooms with cherry tomatoes (*first class, international*)	51	0	1	12%	<1	2%
	Flat iron steak with mushroom butter, eggplant, asparagus, and red bliss mashed potatoes (*first class, international*)	375	74	20	49%	7	17%
	Omelet with bacon, asparagus, and potatoes (*business class, international*)	495	435	35	64%	10	18%
Qantas	Vegetable and bean chili (*first class, domestic*)	260	0	0	0%	0	0%
	Continental breakfast— juice, seasonal melon in fruit syrup, and cereal (*coach, international*)	310	5	3	8%	<1	0%
	Beef fillet, roast potatoes and beans, with anchovy and horseradish						

	Menu item						
	(business class, international)	402	96	15	33%	7	15%
	Marinated lamb cutlets with tzatziki *(first class, domestic)*	356	122	26	66%	11	29%
Scandinavian Airlines	Chili cabbage with rice salad and coconut sauce *(business class)*	377	<1	12	28%	6	14%
	Grilled beef fillet with mashed potatoes, roasted mixed vegetables, and demiglaze sauce *(business class)*	444	68	25	50%	8	17%
Singapore Airlines	Tricolor fettuccine with porcini and portobello mushrooms in herb-tomato sauce *(first/business class, international)*	311	0	5	15%	1	2%
	Roasted bacon–wrapped beef fillet with red wine jus, bone marrow, shallot purée, and sautéed spinach *(first/business class, international)*	451	81	29	58%	10	21%

Nutrition information was estimated from menu item descriptions on airline menus (either provided by the airline or found on the airlines' websites), using the Nutrition Data System for Research v.5.0_35 and Nutrition Analysis Tools and System Version 2.0.

Complimentary meals are still offered in first class on many flights. However, these options are also too high in fat and cholesterol to be considered healthy. An example is the Roasted Double Lamb Chops served on such menus. Fortunately, special meals (including cholesterol-free nondairy vegetarian options) can still be ordered in advance on many flights serving complimentary meals.

Meal service overview: On U.S. and Canadian coach flights that are three hours or longer and depart between 5 A.M. and 9 P.M., a snack box is offered for purchase. On transcontinental, Alaska, and Hawaii flights in coach, a fresh sandwich or wrap is also available for purchase.

Complimentary meal service is provided in coach on Caribbean, Europe, Latin America, Japan, and some Mexico flights that are longer than four hours, within traditional breakfast, lunch, and dinner meal windows. Complimentary food service is offered in first class on all markets systemwide that have flying times over one hour and forty-five minutes and operate within traditional meal (breakfast, lunch, and dinner) windows.

Special meals are available on first- or business-class transcontinental flights in the United States, all classes to and from Europe and Asia, and all classes to and from Rio de Janeiro and São Paulo, Brazil; Buenos Aires, Argentina; Santiago, Chile; and Montevideo, Uruguay.

Continental Airlines
Continental Airlines has hot-meal options for longer domestic flights, but these do not appear to be particularly heart healthy. For example, both the spinach cheese stromboli and the personal cheese pizza are likely to be high in fat and cholesterol. Continental accommodates special requests for overseas and transcontinental flights only, but does not guarantee that all special meals, such as vegan, diabetic, low-fat/low cholesterol, and Hindu, will be available on those flights. Otherwise, no special meals are offered.

Meal service overview: For flights within the United States (over one-and-a-half hours for first class and over two hours for economy class) a complimentary meal or snack is offered on segments during appropriate meal or snack periods. A sandwiches or pizza is the entrée for lunch and dinner. Vegan meals (and other special meals) are available only on certain flights in select markets (mostly international flights or very long domestic flights).

Delta

Delta still offers complimentary domestic meal service, as long as the flight is of a certain distance. Delta's regular meal items usually include some type of healthy side dish such as a mixed green salad or fresh fruit. However, domestic entrée choices leave much to be desired, with such unhealthy options as a cheese omelet served with Canadian bacon at breakfast and a turkey and Swiss cheese sandwich served with potato chips and a cookie as an evening "snack." Travelers on international flights will also find menus filled with high-fat, high-cholesterol items, such as the duck breast with barbecue sauce served with cheese grits or the chicken Caesar salad. Fortunately, travelers can reserve healthier vegan meals in advance.

Meal service overview: Complimentary meal service is available only in first class on flights of 1,550 miles or more and some flights to Hawaii and Alaska and international destinations lasting about five hours or more. When complimentary meal service is available, a special pure vegetarian/vegan meal can be ordered. Snacks are offered on all other flights.

Frontier Airlines

Specifics for menu options were not provided by Frontier, nor can they be found on Frontier's website. Therefore, the PCRM hasn't commented on their healthfulness.

Meal service overview: Frontier offers meals only on long domestic flights (based on distance from Denver) and to Mexico. Meals contain a wrap or a breakfast sandwich (only on flights to Mexico). Specific wrap and breakfast choices were not listed. Snacks are given or sold on some other U.S. flights.

JetBlue
JetBlue is the only airline reviewed by the PCRM that did not provide any in-flight meal, regardless of distance. JetBlue, which is primarily domestic, provides only snack foods such as pretzels, chips, and cookies to their passengers. The airline does, however, allow outside food to be brought on board.

Meal service overview: No meals are provided or sold; only snack foods are available.

Northwest Airlines
Northwest has discontinued its meal service and eliminated special meals on most domestic flights. Travelers can purchase Smartsnacks that mostly look like packaged food products you would find at your local convenience store. Items include cookies and snack crackers, with croissant sandwiches being offered for breakfast. Lunch and dinner Smartsnacks options look better—they include a vegetarian wrap and a vegetarian sandwich. Northwest continues to provide complimentary meals in first class and on international flights, though these are not usually healthy options, and many special meals are no longer offered.

Meal service overview: Snack boxes (Smartsnacks) are available for purchase at meal times in main (coach class) cabin on all domestic flights over 600 miles. In addition, fresh sandwiches are offered in the main cabin on flights to Hawaii, Alaska, and most leisure destinations in Mexico and the Caribbean. Complimentary meal service is still available on some first-class flights. Many special meals have been eliminated.

United Airlines
On United Airlines, fresh food items are available for purchase on many flights of five hours or more. However high-fat and

high-cholesterol options such as the Tuscan Wrap (containing chicken, salami, provolone cheese, and cream cheese spread on a low-carb tortilla) and the Turkey Cobb Salad (containing turkey, Swiss cheese, eggs, and bacon, served with ranch dressing) leave much to be desired.

United also offers SnackBoxes for purchase in economy class on North American flights longer than three-and-a-half hours. These meals are not particularly nutritious, but some do include reasonably healthful items such as unsweetened applesauce and bagel chips.

In addition, complimentary meals are available on some first-class and business-class flights. Breakfast menus offer healthy options such as bagels and breads and a seasonal fruit platter with cereal. Lunch and dinner menus were not reviewed by the PCRM; however, first-class and business-class passengers can request a healthier special meal in advance.

Meal service overview: Complimentary meal service is typically available in first class and business class on flights over two hours that depart during breakfast, lunch, or dinner hours. Special meals, such as vegan meals, are available to these passengers. In economy class, complimentary meals are available on international flights and United p.s. flights between New York's JFK Airport and LAX/SFO in California.

Fresh-food menu items are available for purchase on most North America and Hawaii flights of five hours or longer and on select Mexico and Caribbean flights. SnackBoxes are available for purchase in economy class on North America flights that exceed three-and-a-half hours.

Overseas Airlines

Airlines based overseas typically offer an array of special meals, including healthy vegetarian entrées and options featuring many types of cuisine (Chinese, Indian, Muslim, Western). Some overseas airlines, including Air India and Singapore Airlines, even offer a raw-foods meal. Many also offer healthy options on their regular menus. Air India, British Airways, and Singapore Airlines all seem to offer healthy, plant-based options on a regular basis.

Air China

Many varieties of special meals are available, including three varieties of vegan meals (Western vegan, Eastern vegetarian, and Indian vegan diet). No menus were reviewed by the PCRM.

Air India

First-class, executive-class, and economy-class menus all contain an entire vegetarian menu. The economy-class vegetarian menu contains a Fresh Seasonal Salad, Shak Navratan Korma (a vegetable curry) with Steamed Rice and Dal as the entrée, and Gajar Ka Halwa (carrot pudding) as the dessert.

In addition, a variety of special meals can be ordered, including strict vegetarian, nondairy vegetarian, Asian/Indian vegetarian, and raw vegetarian. This airline seems to be particularly accommodating. According to its website: "Air India takes pride in offering a large variety of meals on board to meet religious or medical requirements or for providing the food you prefer."

Air New Zealand

Although Air New Zealand's sample standard business-class menu does not contain particularly healthy options, the airline takes special care to offer a wide variety of special meals on many of its flights. It offers twenty-two varieties of meals on long-haul flights (e.g., to the United States, United Kingdom, Asia, Perth, Nouméa, or Papeete). For customers traveling on the airline's Tasman or Pacific services, the only special meal offered is a healthy one—a dairy-free vegetarian meal.

British Airways

Dining options are dependent on class: à la carte dining in first class; standard meals in Club World, Club Europe, and World

Traveller classes; and "All Day Deli" meal box in Euro Traveller class.

Special meal requests can be made for all classes except for U.K. domestic flights and Euro Traveller flights. Available healthy options include vegan vegetarian and Asian vegetarian.

First-class menus reviewed included some healthy options. Dinner included two healthy starter options (spicy warm vegetable salad or fresh salad leaves with balsamic vinaigrette), one healthy snack option (penne pasta with tomato and olive ragout), and even a healthy dessert option (fruit). Unfortunately, the main course options were meat-heavy and therefore are not the healthiest choices.

Breakfast in first class also includes some healthy starter options, such as chilled fruit juice and a fresh seasonal fruit plate and rolls from the bakery. Just as with the dinner menu, however, the main-course choices are fat- and cholesterol-laden, such as scrambled eggs served with bacon, pork sausages, sautéed mushrooms, and hash brown potatoes.

First-class brunch likewise doesn't offer a healthy main course option. However, it offers even more healthy starter options, from a fruit plate to tempeh cakes with sweet chili dipping sauce and fresh salad leaves with tomato and basil oil. A healthy snack option (penne pasta with cherry tomato and basil sauce) is also offered on the brunch menu, and fresh fruit is offered as a dessert.

Cathy Pacific

Healthy meal choices on Cathay Pacific are sporadic. In a sample economy-class menu, a healthy supper entrée of penne pasta primavera is offered. However, breakfast options aren't as good, with such choices as an omelet with bacon and fried potatoes. The business- and first-class sample menus reviewed contain no healthy choices for breakfast or supper entrées—only such high-fat options as New York steak and pan-fried halibut served with egg fried rice.

Fortunately, Cathay Pacific offers a variety of special meals, including strict Western vegetarian (vegan), Oriental vegetarian, and strict Indian vegetarian, all of which can be ordered in advance.

Japan Airlines

Healthy meals are very hard to come by on any flights on Japan Airlines. Standard menus for first class, executive class, and economy class were reviewed, and all were very heavy in fatty meat dishes.

One less-than-healthy example is a meal of tandoori chicken, shrimp, salami, and potato salad found on an economy-class dinner menu. Another is a grilled beef fillet with butter, which is offered in the same business-class meal with mayonnaise-laden Waldorf salad. First-class menus make an attempt to note healthy items. However, all of these so-called healthy meals are seafood-based, and therefore contain too much cholesterol to be considered healthy.

As with many of the other airlines, it is important to note that, despite mostly unhealthy standard menus, healthier special meals are available if requested in advance. Special meal choices on Japan Airlines include nonegg, nondairy vegetarian, Asian vegetarian, and raw-foods vegetarian.

Lufthansa

Healthy entrée options were absent from the Lufthansa economy-, business-, and first-class menus reviewed by the PCRM. Some healthy starter options include barley red pepper corn salad with lettuce leaf liner on the economy-class menu, grilled vegetables (portobello mushroom, Japanese eggplant, squash, tomatoes, and asparagus) on the business-class menu, and marinated mushrooms with cherry tomatoes on the first-class menu. If these types of plant-based starters could be translated into entrées, Lufthansa travelers would be much better off.

Lufthansa does take special meal requests; however, a list of specific meal types was not available on their website.

Qantas

Qantas menus do contain some healthy options, but they are few and far between. One first-class menu offers a vegetable-and-bean chili at dinner. A number of side dishes on this menu were healthy as well: fragrant rice, blanched bok choy, char-grilled vegetables, and steamed green beans. Some of the less healthy choices on these same menus are the cream of cauliflower soup with crème fraîche, braised pork sausages, marinated lamb cutlets, and salad of prosciutto, spinach, feta, and walnuts. International business- and economy-class menus did not offer any healthy entrées at lunch or dinner; however, Qantas offers a continental breakfast option that includes juice, seasonal melon in fruit syrup, and cereal.

As with Lufthansa, Qantas apparently allows special meals on request, but a list of these options was not provided on their website.

Scandinavian Airlines (SAS)

Only two business-class menus were reviewed. The vegetarian chili cabbage with rice salad is by far the best choice to be found on these menus, which also include beef fillet and pork tenderloin.

Singapore Airlines

Singapore Airlines offers a "Book the Cook" program to its first- and Raffles- (business-) class passengers. In this program, travelers order their meals before the flight. Unfortunately, only one healthy option is listed here: roasted vegetables with avocado mesclun salad on roesti potatoes.

Healthy options turned up on several standard first- and business-class menus. One notable healthy option was the tricolor fettuccine with porcini and portobello mushrooms in herb-tomato sauce offered at lunch on some flights. If you're lucky enough to be on a flight that offers a vegetarian Indian selection, you'll have multiple healthy choices, such as okra with onion, mushroom and green peas masala, and brown rice.

To be on the safe side, however, since these healthy options are available only on certain flights, health-conscious travelers should call ahead to reserve a vegetarian special meal.

Singapore Airlines was the only airline to provide a children's menu, and, unfortunately, it leaves much to be desired. No healthy, plant-based options are available—only such cholesterol-heavy meals as eggs with sausage and hash browns, fish fingers, spaghetti and meatballs, and macaroni and cheese served with chicken drumlets.

What about special meals? Not surprising, the PCRM recommends trying to preorder these meals when you make your reservations, especially vegetarian choices. However, I need to add an important caution here: In my experience, ordering a special meal and actually having it show up on your flight can be two different experiences. You're still better off bringing your own healthy food on board.

Susan Bowerman, the assistant director for UCLA's Center for Human Nutrition, agrees. Pack your own snacks, especially on short flights, because of the high calorie content (relative to their nutritional value) of the snacks offered by the airlines. "Flying is flying," she says, "and it is not a special event warranting breaking the eating and food rules. It's too easy to make 'special occasions' out of any event, and it's tempting to eat fresh-baked cookies or other high calorie items when they are offered. For people who travel frequently, these extras can add up." And they do.

My biggest challenge, when flying business class on transcon flights, is saying no to the ice cream sundae.

One thing I always do is bring along at least two apples on every flight. Most airline menus are pitifully short on fresh fruit and vegetables. Bowerman says I'm doing the right thing, because fresh fruit and vegetables have the most nutrients and the fewest calories per bite. They provide vitamins, minerals, fiber, phytonutrients, and fluid, and are an important part of the diet.

For years, airlines did their own research on the psychology of in-flight food, and they determined that they had a marketing edge among business travelers if they offered hot breakfasts on early-morning flights. Reason: High-frequency business travelers often looked at airline food as their only opportunity to eat, and if the meal was hot, they felt it had value.

Well, there's perception, and then there's reality.

You need to avoid those hot breakfasts. Why? Many airlines rely on quiches, omelets, French toast, and other calorie-laden dishes, and most people probably don't eat foods this heavy when they are at home. This is a case where coach class may offer better choices, such as high-fiber cereal or yogurt and fruit.

Here are some of Bowerman's other in-flight dining tips: If the airline is offering a sandwich, she recommends taking off the cheese, scraping off any mayonnaise, and then if there was a side salad (since they're usually tiny), she'd probably dump the salad on the sandwich so she wouldn't be tempted to eat the dressing. (My additional salad tip, taught to me by a pilot: On flights where they offer a salad and that little cup of dressing on the side, do *not* pour the dressing on the salad. Instead, dip your fork into the cup, and get a light coating of dressing on it, *then* hit the lettuce.) "Pretzels are better than peanuts in terms of having less fat," Bowerman continues, "but they're still basically a wad of white flour with some salt."

Bowerman also reviewed a selection of airline menus. Following are her findings.

Air Canada

The sample dinner menus are varied and balanced, and do not seem to be as high in fat as those of some other airlines (which rely on sauces, gravies, dressings, and the like and which really rack up calories fast). Fresh-baked cookies will be very tempting. Breakfast menus appear to be quite high in calories and fat (omelets, quiche, meats). Breakfast in any class should focus on lean protein and fruits, such as yogurt plus fruit, high-fiber cereal plus milk and fruit, or if you can get it, some scrambled egg whites with whole grain toast and fruit.

Air India

The menus provided were from first, executive, and coach class. For dinner, fruit is available only in first and executive classes. Generally speaking, Indian food, while delicious, can be deceptively rich. Unless you special-order, it might be difficult to select low-fat items on this airline.

Air New Zealand

This airline has seasonal menus and features local products, which is a nice touch (if you consider local jam and butter to be critical components of your meal). They seem to have an odd definition of "light," however. Dinner on the flight from L.A. to London, for example, includes roasted chicken breast, which would be a healthy choice, but the "light meal" consists of a selection of breads, appetizer of the day, cheese, and chocolate. Similarly, other dinners offer a "light choice" of baked ricotta, Gruyère, and Parmesan tart, which sounds pretty calorie-heavy. The breakfast menu offers a fruit-and-yogurt smoothie, which is great, and also some high-fiber cereals. The hot breakfasts are high in calories and fat, as is true on the other airlines as well. It does not appear that fresh fruit is available for dessert for dinner, which would be nice.

Alaska Airlines

First-class breakfast starts with fruit, which is good—but then again, it is the hot foods (omelet, quiche) that are high in fat and calories. Coach also provides high-fat breakfasts, but has yogurt and fruit, which is the best bet. Entrée salads and side salads are offered in first class, but not in the main cabin, which offers hot sandwiches. Hot sandwiches would need to be deconstructed to make them a little more healthy and could be supplemented with traveler-supplied fruit.

America West

It appears that food is served only in first class. Breakfast, again, can be either reasonable (granola, fruit, milk) or a high-calorie omelet. If grilled chicken or fish is available, that would be a better choice than a casserole-type dish (lasagna, for example). Stay away from the In-Flight Café with its high-calorie, high-fat sandwiches, and from the Fun Box, which has some fruit (fruit bowl, dried cranberries), but the rest is refined carbohydrate snacks (bagel chips, fruit bar, crackers) with a small amount of cheese. The only reasonable choice from the In-Flight Café is the Deli Classic Sandwich, if you remove the cheese. You'd still need to bring fruit or carrots or have a tomato juice to make a reasonably healthy meal.

British Airways

Dinner menus do provide salad (although in my experience on airlines, they are *tiny*). Otherwise, entrées consist of pasta (and generally, pasta entrées on airplanes are heavy and cheesy; this one is no exception) or meat/fish/poultry. Other than the grilled steak, they appear to be heavy and high in fat. The desserts are rich and should be avoided.

Cathay Pacific

With its emphasis on Chinese cuisine but with accommodations for Western palates, this menu could provide some of the more healthy dishes in the air. Fruit and yogurt are available for breakfast, as well as cereal (not high-fiber, but at least they are alternatives to the other high-fat items available). This is not offered in economy class, where you can get an omelet, seafood congee, or banana bread. Even in economy class, the Asian-inspired entrées are lighter than the Western-style entrées.

Continental
Here you face the same issues with the hot breakfast entrées; opt for fruit or cereal whenever they are available. In economy class, the lunch and dinner selections are hot or cold sandwiches. If this is all that is available, remove the cheese from the sandwiches if you can. They do offer baby carrots, fruit, and a small salad with the sandwiches, which is good.

Frontier Airlines
This airline does not give out enough information to go on. Muffins, pretzels, snack baskets, and cookies are not exactly cornerstones of a healthy diet. The same goes for the breakfast sandwiches.

Hawaiian Airlines
Here's an interesting twist: Coach class offers a salad to start, as opposed to baby greens with a warm goat cheese tart in first class. Most other airlines don't even offer salad in coach. One thing to keep in mind with salads is that they are generally served with dressing on the side, so you can control how much you use. First-class entrées appear to offer enough selection that you could choose something healthy, such as grilled fish or chicken breast, but in coach it's pasta again or possibly a sandwich. The Hawaiian plate is a bad choice: teriyaki chicken with rice and potato macaroni salad! Not a fruit or vegetable to be seen. And you get coffee ice cream on top of it!

Japan Airlines

These menus, for the most part, are great. With emphasis on healthy Japanese cuisine, there are an abundance of choices. Chicken, fish, salads, and fruits are available across the board, at least in first class and business class. Coach lunches and dinners have some light items available as entrées, and breakfast can include fruit and yogurt, as well as tea. Again, Western-style entrées (pasta dishes) tend to be higher in fat, and Western-type breakfasts should also be avoided.

JetBlue

This is a great airline, but when it comes to food, it's nothing short of a snacking disaster. Bring your own. Cookies, chips, pretzels . . . who needs them?

Lufthansa

As with the others, choices in first and business class are a little more imaginative, and offer a few more fruits, vegetables, and salads. The economy-class sample menu includes a meat entrée and a pasta entrée, which seems to be the way most of the airlines go in order to offer a vegetarian choice for those who do not preorder. The breakfast box does get away from the hot meals, and a sandwich can be modified (remove the cheese) and consumed with the fruit yogurt that is provided, for a reasonably well-balanced meal. Skipping the bars and the shortbread biscuits and carrying your own fruit would be the healthy approach. It appears that only first class offers nonfat yogurt with fresh fruit or cereal and milk.

Northwest Airlines

No coach-class information was available. The first-class menus look a lot like coach menus on other airlines (sandwich plate with chips and potato salad), probably because they do not have as many long flights. So on a flight of three hours or less, passengers should ask themselves if they really need to eat. Carrying your own healthy snacks of fruits, vegetables, a healthier sandwich, or a protein bar would be a much better bet than purchasing the snack boxes or premade sandwiches offered here.

Qantas

Qantas does an innovative thing, at least in first class. You can customize your meals at dinner by selecting your own side dishes to go with your main course. In the sample menu given, three of the six choices were vegetables, so you could make quite a healthy dinner for yourself by avoiding some of the higher-fat, higher-calorie starches. Sliced fresh seasonal fruit is also a dessert choice that is rarely seen on any airline menu.

Southwest

High-calorie snack packs. Enough said.

Swissair

Salads, grilled meats, fish, and poultry are available (as is the case in first class on most airlines). Yogurt and fruit are available for breakfast. Swiss chocolate is probably something worth saving your calories for.

United Airlines

In terms of the snack box selections, opt for the Jumpstart, only because it has a fruit bowl, fruit-and-nut mix, and green tea. Avoid the Wheat Thins and probably the sunflower seed spread, and forgo the granola bar. The Mini Meal is very high in fat, with cheese spread, hard salami, potato chips, and Milano cookies.

US Air

In-Flight Café meals: Both breakfasts offer fresh fruit; one entrée consists of ham and cream cheese on raisin bread; the other is a blueberry loaf served with yogurt. Again, you could do a lot better bringing your own fruit, a protein bar, a carton of light yogurt, or a small amount of trail mix. The lunch sandwich available for purchase is high in fat and is served with chips and a cookie—also very high in fat and calories.

TO DRINK OR NOT TO DRINK

We've already mentioned that you should avoid alcoholic beverages preflight. This goes for alcohol on the plane as well. There are a number of really good reasons why you should never drink on a flight. Nevertheless, people continue to ask for a drink during their flight. And the airlines continue to stock lots of alcohol. American Airlines, for example, maintains fifteen different wine lists for passengers in first and business class. The airline purchases 260,000 cases of wine a year. At any given time, American has more than sixty wines in the air.

Airlines take their wine seriously. The man who selects wines for American is named Richard Vine (yes, that's his real name), a retired Purdue University professor of enology. The airline might lose your bags, it might not be on time, and it *will* charge for meals in coach, but you can count on American to change its wine list monthly, posting a thirty-eight-page pamphlet online that describes each route's selections in detail. Each wine list includes two reds, two whites, a champagne, a dessert wine, and sometimes a sherry. Flights to Asia add a pair of sake selections.

Considering all that effort by American and some other airlines to offer varied wine selections, it's too bad that, like food, wine tastes different in flight. At 35,000 feet, the sense of smell is dulled, making subtle flavors nearly impossible to detect. (For that reason, airline wine selections tend to be on the bold side to have impact.)

Whether or not the wine selection is the reason, I continue to be amazed by the number of my friends who drink on their flights. Even worse, some of them drink alcohol in conjunction with prescription drugs like Ambien and Lunesta.

The one thing you should *always* drink on a plane is water—and a lot of it. Here are some interesting facts about water.

Some 75 percent of us are chronically dehydrated (and that's *before* we get on a plane). Here's the worst part: According to one recent study, in 37 percent of Americans, the thirst mechanism is so weak that it is often mistaken for hunger. And one more thing: Even mild dehydration will slow down your metabolism by as much as 3 percent. Conversely, in one German study, researchers looked at the caloric intake and energy expenditure of men and women who consumed two glasses of water a day. The studies revealed that within ten minutes of drinking the water, the metabolic rate increased by a staggering 30 percent.

So if you want to lose weight and you travel, you should drink tons of water.

UCLA's Susan Bowerman advises drinking about 8 ounces of noncaffeinated fluid for every hour you are in the air. Not only will it hydrate you, but it will also curb your appetite. However, there's *one huge warning here.* Don't drink the water that's *on* the plane. This is nonnegotiable. BYO.

And that even includes flights where you see the flight attendants serving bottled water. Why? Read on. It's not pretty.

WELCOME TO THE WORLD OF . . . TAPPIAN

I'm not impressed anymore when I see a flight attendant serving water on a flight. But I am concerned. Where did that water come from?

Just ask the Environmental Protection Administration. In the summer of 2004, the EPA tested drinking water aboard 327

U.S. and foreign flag aircraft at nineteen airports. The agency did water-quality sampling on galley water taps, water fountains, and lavatory faucets. The results were not pleasant: The data showed that 13 percent of tested aircraft water failed to meet EPA standards and tested positive for the presence of total coliform bacteria. They tested again in the fall, and the results were even worse: Seventeen percent failed the standards.

As a result, the EPA announced consent orders with eleven major domestic airlines and thirteen smaller and low-cost airlines to implement new aircraft water testing and disinfection protocols.

Administrative orders on consent have been finalized with the following airlines:

AirTran Airways	Miami Air International
Alaska Airlines	Midwest Airlines
Aloha Airlines	North American Airlines
American Airlines	Northwest Airlines
America West	Pace Airlines
ATA	Ryan International Airlines
Champion Air	Spirit Airlines
Continental Airlines	Sun Country Airlines
Continental Micronesia	United Airlines
Falcon Air Express	US Airways
Frontier Airlines	USA 3000 Airlines
Hawaiian Airlines	World Airways

The administrative orders on consent require the airlines to implement regular monitoring and disinfection protocols for their entire fleet of aircraft for a period of two years. Specifically, the orders require the airlines to perform regular monitoring of aircraft water systems, regularly disinfect aircraft water systems and water transfer equipment, undertake corrective action and provide public notice when there is a total coliform positive sample result, and conduct a study of possible sources of contamination that exist outside of the aircraft.

But now, let's look at the specifics of the order: The airlines are required to provide total coliform and disinfectant residual samples from at least one galley and lavatory on every aircraft in a twelve-month time period. Just once in a twelve-month period? That's not encouraging.

Does this EPA report and the consent agreements mean it's now OK to drink the water on planes? No way. These EPA agreements do not include any penalties. They are just administrative orders based on the consent of the airlines themselves. They assume good faith. My response: *Good luck.*

Even the EPA, while announcing these agreements with airlines to further inspect their water, issued the following disclaimer:

Passengers with suppressed immune systems or others concerned should request bottled or canned beverages while on the aircraft and refrain from drinking tea or coffee that does not use bottled water. While boiling water for one minute will remove pathogens from drinking water, the water used to prepare coffee and tea aboard a plane is not generally brought to a sufficiently high temperature to guarantee that pathogens are killed.

But there's something even worse: In the United States, water loaded aboard aircraft comes from public water systems. The water provided by public water systems is regulated by state and federal authorities. That water may be delivered to the aircraft holding tank via pipes from the airport itself or using a hose from a water tanker. But with international flights, all bets are off. A majority of these aircraft get water from foreign sources not subject to EPA drinking water standards.

OK, now let's do the math. One in six airplanes flying today is flying with unsafe drinking water.

My qualified advice: Drink bottled water. Why qualified? Because even with bottled water, there's a problem on airplanes. And again, it's not pretty. While a number of airlines now stock bottled water on their flights, they don't stock enough. And very soon after takeoff, flight attendants often find that they've run out of water. That's when it gets dicey. What do they do? They simply refill the empty water bottles from the galley supply (the airline's holding tanks), and that's when people get sick. The flight attendants call this water . . . "tappian."

The simple solution here: Bring a half dozen 8-ounce bottles of water with you on every flight. As I've said, the water will not only hydrate you but curb your appetite. You won't eat airline food (or much of it), and you won't get sick.

SOME FINAL ADVICE FOR THE PLANE TRIP

Here's my advice on how you should spend your time on planes: sleep, work or read, and move around.

The sleep part is easy, and despite the placement and size of my seat and how crowded the flight is, I still usually manage to get some quality work done. It's the moving around part that's the challenge. But you must do it, for an important health reason.

Deep vein thrombosis, or DVT, is sometimes called "economy-class syndrome" thanks to its association with the lack of legroom for long-haul coach passengers. Despite that fairly innocuous-sounding name, DVT is a serious medical condition that can, if not prevented or treated, be fatal.

DVT occurs when a blood clot forms, usually in the leg, as a result of poor circulation. DVT is often seen in patients who've undergone major surgery and have poor or no mobility as a result. While DVT can cause swelling, pain, and discomfort, the real threat is if, and/or when, this clot breaks free and travels to the lungs. This results in a pulmonary embolism, which, if untreated, can be fatal within hours. Although the chance of a dramatic collapse and death from a pulmonary embolism while in flight or after disembarking is only one in one million travelers, DVT strikes more than one in one thousand adults each year and is worth preventing.

The major controllable risk factors associated with DVT include anything that can inhibit proper circulation, such as lack of exercise, smoking, and being overweight. Heavier people are at risk because the blood in their legs doesn't circulate as much and tends to pool there.

There are a number of other factors, less easy to control, that increase an individual's risk for DVT. These include a family history of DVT or pulmonary embolisms, estrogen usage or pregnancy, and vein disease.

The good news about DVT is that, for most people, it's fairly easy to prevent, as long as you remain aware of your circumstances.

Dr. Samuel Z. Goldhaber, a cardiologist at Brigham and Women's Hospital in Boston, who has specialized in DVT for over twenty-five years, says one of the best ways to prevent DVT is to stay well hydrated. "Take your own personal stash of water on the plane and drink enough to get up and go to the bathroom and urinate. Walking forces the blood to circulate in the deep leg veins." Dehydration causes the blood cells to become thicker and clottable, so drinking water helps to keep blood thinner. Avoid alcohol, which can be dehydrating. Wearing vascular compression stockings also keeps blood flowing through veins if the stockings are fitted properly.

And be sure to stand up and walk around—once per hour should be sufficient. When you do get up to move around, stretch your calf muscles by standing on your toes several times to increase your circulation.

DVT is a very serious medical condition, but if you begin to have symptoms of DVT, don't panic. The good news is that most airports have medical facilities, and even if you're flying into a particularly underdeveloped place, medical care will be available near, or sometimes at, nearly all airports. The bad news is that DVT often has few or no symptoms at all. And, as Goldhaber points out, sometimes it takes days for symptoms to develop. "You might begin feeling an ache or cramp in the calf several days after traveling. The blood clot could have started on the plane and not be discovered until weeks later. It's important to remain vigilant." Often DVT feels like a cramp or charley horse in the lower part of the leg that simply doesn't get better.

These are the most common symptoms of DVT:

- Cramping or aching in the leg, particularly when moved

- Elevated skin temperature in the area

- Surface veins that become particularly noticeable

- Swelling of the feet and legs

Long-term ways of preventing DVT include adopting a healthy lifestyle with good nutrition, maintaining a lean body weight, and engaging in a regular exercise program.

Forty thousand new cases of DVT and pulmonary embolism are diagnosed in the United States each year. No one knows how many undetected cases there are for every detected case. The ratio may be three to five undetected cases for every detected case, which could mean one to two million new cases every year.

But remember, while DVT is a serious disease, it is largely preventable. Whether you're a frequent flier or just an occasional one, it pays to be aware of the risks and symptoms of this disease. If you're at high risk of DVT, because of either the frequency of your travels or the risk factors noted here, it would be a good idea to talk to your doctor about treatment and prevention options for your particular circumstances.

The Absurdity of In-Flight Yoga and Exercise

I am sure it is absolutely well-intentioned. In principle, it's a great idea. And over the years a number of airlines, from SAS to Song have offered in-flight exercise and fitness programs.

Most recently, an in-flight fitness program designed by fitness guru David Barton was launched on all Song flights. As part of its in-flight fitness program, the airline sold a resistance band, a ball, and an easy-to-follow workout booklet for $8, for an in-seat workout you could do on the plane or in your hotel room. The program utilized "resistance tube training for increasing strength, core abdominal work for maintaining postural integrity and dynamic release for stimulating blood and relieving tension knots." By the end of 2005, Song had sold out of this product three times (15,000 packages) and hopes to incorporate the program on its Delta flights.

However, there is a drawback: The people who bought the program couldn't really exercise in flight without injuring—or at least severely annoying—their seatmate (or both).

Swissair, Qantas, and Australian Air also offer in-flight exercise ideas on their websites, but I have yet to see a single passenger following those ideas on any flights I've ever taken.

JetBlue and Crunch Fitness International joined forces to design an Airplane Yoga and Airplane Pilates program to help you stretch and relax while you are flying. A Crunch Fitness Airplane Yoga card was available in the seatback pocket on all JetBlue flights starting in 2002, giving passengers an illustrated guide to unobtrusive yoga positions.

But again, there were problems. You really needed to alert someone on the plane before you started doing this, because the program required you to repeatedly stretch upward with both hands, which could be alarming to other passengers as well as to flight attendants. It didn't take long for the JetBlue instruction sheet to offer a caution: "A flight attendant may ask you if you need something. Tell them that we all need inner peace . . ."

Perhaps that's why, in 2004, the JetBlue airplane yoga program evolved into a Pilates program.

And now, I'll offer one. It won't cost you anything. Once the seat belt sign is off and the beverage carts are out of the aisles, get out of your seat and walk around the plane. Stretch in the small spaces between cabins or in the companionways near lavatories. And if you can't, for whatever reason, do that, then focus on muscle isolation exercises in your seat. This involves isometric tightening of your muscles and is perhaps easiest to do while seated, since this technique uses very small movements. It's actually quite simple. Just sit straight up and take a deep breath. Then, as you exhale, you can tighten your stomach muscles and simply hold for a count of 20. Then release and repeat ten times. Do this once every thirty minutes or so (in between drinking those 8-ounce bottles of water you brought with you), and you can choose a different muscle group to work with each time.

Then switch to your legs (and if you can do this on an economy flight, in a coach seat, you win an additional prize from me). In this exercise, with your feet flat on the floor, raise one leg a few inches. Hold the position for thirty seconds. Repeat with the other leg. There are shoulder and biceps exercises as well, but, trust me, they are too awkward, and look too embarrassing, for me to recommend.

My best advice: Again, walk around and stretch on the plane. Because the real exercise awaits you—at your hotel.

CHAPTER 5

At the Hotel: Eating

As I have learned in researching this book, the real battleground for the traveler's diet is not in the air—it's on the ground, once we land and check in at our hotel. It's sad but true: Hotels and resorts are where all good diet and health intentions go to die. The culprit is a lethal combination of food, sleep deprivation, and lack of exercise.

When it comes to diet, exercise, and fitness on the road, we are indeed a nation in denial.

As soon as we arrive at a hotel, our self-control seems to evaporate. Whether it's a business trip or a vacation, we're operating on different schedules, in different environments, exposed to different climates, cultures, foods. As a result, we pack on the pounds.

More often than not, we are eating out. In 1955, Americans spent 19 percent of their food dollar on food that was prepared outside the home. Today it's nearing 50 percent, and climbing. Not only do we eat out more often, but invariably, when we eat out, the portions are larger. And we're cleaning our plates. You do the math . . .

That's the way it was with me. Not only was I eating at odd hours, but my frequency of eating increased and the amounts were getting larger. Exercise wasn't even part of the deal. And what I was eating was enough to make my original food diary look like I was training for the Tour de France. But it doesn't have to be that way.

Simple adjustments make the difference. Let's look at the way most people travel. They arrive at their hotel—after being abused by airports and airlines—and it's late. They're tired; they walk into their room, take off their shoes, turn on the TV, stare at the minibar, order a burger and fries from room service, log on to the Internet immediately, and then sleep poorly.

Translation: Arriving at your hotel is the beginning of the end of your diet.

And in my case, I didn't even wait for room service. I was the king of the one-two *munch*. Even as room service was processing my order—and as much as I despise the minibar—it's amazing how quickly I would justify the outrageous cost of a Snickers at 11:30 at night. Greenberg Axiom #1: If you look at that Snickers bar long enough, you are going to eat it. Elasticity of desire, at least in my case, was in direct proportion to the elasticity of my waistline.

So, to stay fit on the road, it's important to enlist the hotel on your side.

Call ahead and ask that the minibar be either locked or removed altogether. There is a third alternative: On your way to the hotel, have the cab pull over at a nearby supermarket. Go in and buy bottled water and lots of fruit. When you arrive at the hotel, ask them to empty the minibar. Then you can restock it with your own healthy choices. (In hotels that have installed the new, draconian Darth Vader minibars—the ones with infrared sensors that charge you if you even touch a Diet Coke—ask the housekeeping staff to bring you a small refrigerator. Many hotels have these available for guests' use.

Perhaps most important, we all need to recognize that we really don't change our lifestyles when we change our location. And business travelers (with few exceptions) are extreme creatures of habit.

We need to disrupt those patterns. I know I had to do that. And it was surprisingly easy for me to do it.

My travel patterns allowed it. I don't check bags; I FedEx them. Not only am I saving time during the actual travel process (no schlepping of bags to and from airports, no baggage carousels, and no waiting), but I save time when I arrive at the hotel, since in many cases my bags are already in my

room. So the check-in process is relatively smooth and seam-
less.

Now, instead of doing a traditional hotel check-in, where I
show up at the front desk, show my credit card, get my keys, and
go to my room, I interrupt that process: I've called ahead, I'm
met at the front desk by a trainer from the hotel's gym, and I'm
taken immediately to the health club for a one-hour workout.
(Much more on this in Chapter 6.)

Then there's the hotel food itself. Most hotels these days—
especially the larger chains—have begun to embrace the concept,
if not the execution, of a healthier menu at their restaurants. But
that still doesn't mean that we eat healthier, or know how to
order healthier, when we're on the road.

It all comes down to a definition of the word *healthy,* and how
precise you are when you order the food. Certain hotels try to
help. Hilton offers its Eat Right menu, which is a separate menu
of healthy eating options. Radisson is in the testing phase of its
Tasteful Choice menu, for which it is developing sixteen overall
healthy and light dishes with the Culinary Institute of America in
California's Napa Valley. A few years ago, Starwood rolled out a
low-carb menu. It looked good in theory, but was a miserable failure. Only 3 percent of the guests ordered from that menu.

Marriott's Fit for You menus get very specific. They offer
designated dishes that correlate to different types of diets: carb-
conscious, low-cholesterol, and low-fat. These dishes appear
with stars on the menu, for easy identification. Many of the
dishes are broken down according to their calorie, fat, protein,
and carbohydrate content. For an item to be designated as
"healthy," it has to adhere to certain guidelines, containing no
more than:

- 19.5 grams of fat

- 6.0 grams of saturated fat

- 90 milligrams of cholesterol

- 720 milligrams of sodium

"We rolled out the plan," says Robin Uler, who oversees all the Marriott food offerings, "because we have found through research that while we say we'll cook anything, many people are hesitant to ask, so we found that if we identified something as low cholesterol, people would order it."

Perhaps most important, Uler has incorporated the main Fit for You menu into the kids' menu, adding grilled chicken strips and fresh fruit. And not a moment too soon: Wisconsin researchers recently studied 621 children in one school district and discovered that school-age kids who ate out four or more times a week showed increases in blood pressure, bad cholesterol counts, and weight gain. After all, eating at hotels is eating out.

So everyone at Marriott is eating healthier? Of course not. What people say they do and what they really do at hotels are two very different things. No matter how healthy the menu offerings at the hotel, if a Pizza Hut is nearby, the call will be made.

Like Marriott, a separate healthier menu is now a brand standard at two hundred Hilton hotels, including Embassy Suites and DoubleTree, and it is appropriately called Eat Right. In preparation for the program, Hilton chefs attended an intense five-day training course at Johnson & Wales University. Then they created the menus, including more than one hundred recipes that incorporate grains, fruits, and vegetables and use a limited amount of saturated fats and cholesterol, along with moderate amounts of sugar and sodium.

These Eat Right menus provide a complete breakdown for each item, in milligrams, of carbs, fat, sodium, and protein, and they tell you the total amount of calories in each dish. Guests can even go online to the Flavors of Hilton website (accessed via Hilton.net), where along with the nutritional facts, the hotel of-

fers the complete, downloadable recipes for menu items—
everything from Ahi Tuna and Grilled Salmon to Citrus Grilled
Chicken Breast. There's even a Kentucky Onion Ribeye with a
glaze that meets the healthy criteria. Overseas, Hilton International has its own Healthy Options program available in more
than eighty hotels in Europe and Africa. No dish on this menu
contains more than 400 calories.

In spite of all these well-intentioned attempts at healthy
menus, it's nevertheless absolutely necessary that you decon-
struct your meal.

"Just because an item is starred as a healthy choice means
nothing," says Anthony Scotto, whose family owns and operates
Fresco, one of my favorite restaurants in Manhattan. "You see
the salmon or the swordfish on the menu and it's got that aster-
isk," he says. "And that's supposed to mean that they will cook it
without butter or heavy sauces." The reality, he says, is often very
different. "Back in the kitchen, there's one guy on the line and
his only job is cooking fish. And he's cooking all of it the same
way." Scotto's advice: Unless you have a great relationship with a
restaurant owner or individual chef, assume nothing. You must
construct your meal by deconstructing it ahead of time. "Order
the fish dry, not the way it's listed on the menu," he advises. "You
can even order the sauce on the side and be responsible for minimum amounts."

Scotto is right. I've tried this at a number of hotel restaurants, and the difference is immediately noticeable—and so is
the calorie and fat count.

Furthermore, menu language likewise has to be deconstructed. So I asked a number of hotel chefs and dieticians to analyze hotel menus and suggest healthy choices from them. I
omitted the hotel name from the menus that I showed them, des-
ignating them by a letter-and-number code (the actual restaurant
names appear in parentheses here). First up is Achim Lenders,
executive chef at Hyatt, with his conclusions about these menus.

Menu A1 (Wyndham Tremont House, Boston)

Overall, the menu looks very rich and the dishes use a lot of preparation methods and ingredients that are heavy in fat and calories. The salads look healthy; however, ask for the dressings to be served on the side. Stay away from all cream or butter sauces, or ask for the dishes to be served plain, with the sauces on the side.

Menu A2 (Wyndham, Toledo)

This menu is healthier and offers lower-calorie choices. Ask for the sauces to be served on the side. Substitute seeds or nuts for bacon. Remove cheese from some of the choices. Choose the Garlic and Herb Roasted Chicken or the Grilled Salmon Fillet from the entrées.

Menu B1 (InterContinental San Francisco, Nob Hill)

These are very clearly laid out and labeled choices. The items are healthy and low in calories. Some of the vegetarian items are high in calories and fat. Any of the healthy choices would be good.

Menu B2 (InterContinental, Montreal)

The menu is very Mediterranean and is generally healthy. This chef uses a lot of reductions and items that are sweet-and-sour to create an interesting menu. All the dishes are prepared with minimal fat and should be low in calories.

Menu C1 (Hilton, Omaha)

All dishes are clearly labeled with the amount of fats, carbohydrates, and calories, which makes it easy to choose. Somehow it takes the fun out of the eating . . .

Menus D1 and D2 (DoubleTree, Roanoke and San Jose)

The menus are designed for the health-conscious traveler. D2 has some dishes with more than 800 calories; this is a lot for one dish, considering that the average intake should be around 2,800 calories per day for an active man. This dish represents around 30 percent of the daily intake, without accounting for beverages and the like. The total amount of calories consumed for a day should not exceed the recommended daily intake.

Menus E1 and E2 (Embassy Suites, Milpitas and Atlanta)

All dishes are clearly labeled with the amount of fats, carbohydrates, and calories, which makes it easy to choose. Somehow it takes the fun out of the eating . . .

Menu F1 (Park Hyatt—Sambar, Goa)

Although vegetarian, this menu is not very healthy. Most of the Indian dishes use a lot of butter and other animal fats in the preparation of dals and curries—tandoori dishes would be good choices.

Menus G1 and G2 (Marriot, Redmond, Washington, and Vancouver)

Items are clearly labeled, however, some of the low carb dishes use carbohydrates-rich ingredients like linguini or barley risotto. Overall the menu appears to be well balanced and offers a lot of choices.

Menus H1 and H2 (Westin, Grand Cayman and St. Louis)

The healthy choices of H1 are not very interesting—just vegetables with some dressing. They look more like vegetarian items. H2's items are more interesting, but one of them uses Brie cheese, which is high in fat.

I also asked Marriott's nutritional consultant to evaluate some of the same, as well as some additional, anonymous hotel menus.

Menu A1 (Wyndham Tremont House, Boston)

Try to avoid the Caesar salad unless you ask for the dressing on the side. Dressing tends to be high in cholesterol and fat. Seafood Au Gratin is not a good choice because of the cream sauce. The best choices are the Tremont House Salad and the Roasted Vegetable Stacks. The best choice if you are considering a low-fat salad is the Fresh Atlantic Salmon Salad, if dressing is served on the side. Salmon tends to be high in fat, but it is good fat in the form of omega-3 fatty acids. This consultant also recommends the Chicken Piñata (ask for the Lemon Butter Caper Sauce on the side) and the Pan-Seared Red Snapper because it is made with vegetable broth, as opposed to a dish with a cream base. The Seafood Gumbo would be a good alternative to the snapper dish. Both entrées have positives and negatives. The gumbo contains sausage, which would be higher in fat, but the snapper is served with goat cheese and mashed potatoes. The rest of the entrées would be good choices if the sauces were served on the side. The best carb-conscious dish would be the New York Strip Steak.

Menu B1 (InterContinental San Francisco, Nob Hill)

The choices marked healthy on this menu seem to be in line, for the most part. The Grilled Ahi Tuna would be lower in fat, cholesterol, and carbohydrates. The prix fixe dinner is a three-course meal in which the Grilled Swordfish would be the best choice. Duck tends to be high in fat.

B2 Heart Healthy (InterContinental, Montreal)

Most of the appetizers are good choices. The Grilled Eggplant Stuffed with Walnuts is higher in fat, but it's a good fat, so it would be a good choice. The best choice among the main courses would be the Grilled Chicken Breast Poached in Vegetable Stock (ask for the yogurt sauce on the side). Mediterranean-style dishes would also be good choices, but, again, ask for the cream tomato sauce on the side.

Menu C1 (Hilton, Omaha)

A good choice here is the Tarragon Chicken Salad with Arugula, to lower the fat and cholesterol, but eliminate the hard-boiled eggs—there is enough protein in the chicken.

Menu C2 (Hilton, Waikoloa Village)

Choose the Smoked Chicken Linguine for a low-fat meal. The best carb-conscious choice is the Shrimp Cobb Salad if the dressing is served on the side.

Menus D1 and D2 (DoubleTree, Roanoke)

The best choice would be the Pepper Tuna with Cucumber Fennel Salad, and the second choice would be Mediterranean Grilled Chicken Salad, but ask for the dressing on the side. Both of these would also be good carb-conscious options.

Menu D2 (DoubleTree, San Jose)

The best low-fat choice is the Grilled Chicken Breast. The best carb-conscious dish is the Tropical Shrimp Cobb Salad. To reduce the fat, ask for the dressing on the side.

Menu E1 (Embassy Suites, Milpitas–Silicon Valley)

The best choice here is the Grilled Free-Range Chicken, and the Pan-Seared Asian Tuna Salad would be a good second choice, but ask for the dressing on the side.

Menu E2 (Embassy Suites, Atlanta Airport)

The Sautéed Chicken Salad is the best choice. Adding the Cold Cucumber Soup would make a nice meal.

Menu F1 (Park Hyatt—Sambar, Goa)

Coconut milk tends be high in fat, so avoid dishes made with this ingredient. The menu had numerous selections, but here are some recommendations: Sambar Tomato Pappu (dal), Chetti-nadu Kozhi Curry, Chapala Pulusu (a fish stew), and Soppu Palya (a spinach and lentil curry). The best low-carb meal would be the Sprouts and Vegetable Salad.

Menu F2 (Grand Hyatt, New York)

The best sandwich is the Roasted Turkey Breast, with Avocado Aioli on the side. The best entrée is the French Cut Chicken Breast and Saffron Vegetable Risotto. The best salad is the Marinated Grilled Chicken Salad.

Menu H1 (Westin, Grand Cayman)

The Organic Garden Salad and Baby Greens are both good choices if the dressing is served on the side. Roasted Turkey Club and Grilled Free-Range Chicken sandwiches are also good options if the mayonnaise is served on the side. Substitute fresh fruit for fries.

Among the entrées, the first choice would be the Vegetarian Penne Pasta. The next-best choice would be a low-carb dish—Caribbean Farfalle with Spicy Chicken, but ask for the cream sauce on the side.

Menu H2 (Westin—Clark Street Grill, St. Louis)

The Certified Angus Beef Grill with Teriyaki Flat Steak is marked as nutritionally balanced for calories, cholesterol, and fat. However, a beef or steak meal is not generally a good choice. The Savory Cabbage Roulades would be a better choice. The Penne Pasta would also be a good choice if a tomato-type sauce was substituted for the cream sauce. If the Plantain-Crusted Mahimahi is not fried but stir-fried, this would be a good choice as well. Garlic and Herb Roasted Chicken is OK if the skin is removed. The customer should do this at the table because it is best to cook the chicken in the skin to retain the moisture. Another acceptable choice is the Stuffed Flounder, with the sauce served on the side.

If you order a sandwich, replace the fries with a small green salad, with dressing on the side. Recommendations for sandwiches are the Southwestern Shrimp Wrap, with guacamole on the side, and the Sheraton Club Sandwich without the bacon, and with dressing on the side. The Mexican City Caesar Salad is also a good choice if dressing is served on the side.

Menu I2 (Sheraton, Puerto Rico)

Good choices are the Grilled Ajillo Shrimp Skewers and the Fire Roasted Spiced Ahi Tuna.

To make a carb-conscious meal, order a side of mushrooms or mixed steamed vegetables. Avoid the Saffron Roasted Potatoes, rice and beans, and garbanzos if you are striving for a carb-conscious option. Also avoid the creamed spinach if you are going for a low-fat option. The best choices from among the sauce offerings would be the Rum Peppercorn Sauce and the Smoky Island Barbecue Sauce.

Menu J1 (Four Seasons, Costa Rica)

Calzones tend to be high in fat. The best pizza is the Wild Mushroom, but removing the bacon is recommended. The best low-fat offerings are the Corn Crusted Mahimahi, but grilled rather than fried, and the Tamarine Crusted Ahi Tuna. When a dish is listed as "crusted," it's a good idea to ask how it is prepared.

Menu J2 (Four Seasons, Boston)

A good choice here is the Spaghetti Caprese or the Hybrid Bass. Salmon would be another good choice, although it tends to be higher in cholesterol and fat, but then again, it contains good omega-3 fatty acids. On the side, Grilled Asparagus or wild mushrooms would be the best choice.

Menu K1 (Ritz-Carlton, Marina Del Rey)

Here, the best appetizers are the Sizzling Wasabi Shrimp and the Chicken Yakitori. Among entrées, choose the Hawaiian Swordfish or the French Sea Bass, which is a good carb-conscious meal if only a small amount of the corn is consumed. For cold starters, try the Homemade Tofu and the Heirloom Salad.

Menu K2 (Ritz-Carlton, Lake Las Vegas)

For the first course, try the Mixed Baby Green Salad, with dressing on the side. For the second course, order the Hawaiian Prawns or the Atlantic Salmon, if the citrus butter is served on the side. Again, the salmon contains good omega-3 fatty acids but will be higher in fat and cholesterol.

Menu L1 (Kimpton, Vancouver)

A good carb-conscious dish here is the Butter Curry Scallops, but ask them to go light on the butter sauce. As a second choice, try the Mole Tuna.

Menu M1 (Radisson, Northbrook)

Select the Willows Green Salad, with dressing on the side, to accompany the swordfish main dish. A good second choice would be the salmon. The Shrimp and Scallop Farfalle will work if the sauce is served on the side.

Menu M2 (Radisson, Winnipeg)

Recommended dishes here include the Atlantic Salmon, Connie's Stir-Fry (vegetables tossed in black bean sauce and sesame oil over a bed of rice), and Penne Pasta, with sauce on the side— pesto sauces tend to be higher in fat.

Next, I asked Cynthia Sass, of the ADA, to analyze the same menus. The following chart summarizes her findings.

	InterContinental	Hilton	DoubleTree	Embassy Suites	Marriott	Westin	Sheraton	Kimpton
Overall Positives	Heart symbol indicates "healthy" selections (however, no explanation provided of criteria for symbol). Good menu variety. Vegetarian options available.	Calorie and nutrition facts information provided!	This was confusing because the analysis of the recipes was here, but is this available to the customer? It looks like they also use the Hilton Eat Right menus as per the nutrition labels, but the information isn't listed under each menu item as it is on the Hilton menus. Also, there was an analysis of only some of the menu items, not all.	Calorie and nutrition facts information provided!	Fit for You symbol indicates special selections, including low-carb, low-cholesterol, and low-fat (however, no explanation provided of criteria for each). Vegetarian options available.	Sun (is that what it is?) symbol indicates Health Smart selections (however, no explanation provided of criteria for this symbol). Some vegetarian options available	I'm at a loss for words here – this menu is peppered with nutritional land mines.	This isn't quite as bad as Sheraton, but this is also a challenging menu. There are some good seafood options, but if you're allergic or don't like seafood, it will be difficult to stay light here.

	InterContinental	**Hilton**	**DoubleTree**	**Embassy Suites**	**Marriott**	**Westin**	**Sheraton**	**Kimpton**
Overall Negatives	No calorie or nutrition facts information. The prix fixe dinner is quite decadent!	None! This is fantastic!	No nutrition facts listed under each menu item. No portion size information provided — e.g., is the smoothie 8 ounces or 20 ounces, is the salmon 4 ounces or 12 ounces? Also, fairly limited menu — just one page.	None! This is fantastic!	No calorie or nutrition facts information on menu. (Possibly available upon request?) Many rich menu selections.	No calorie or nutrition facts information on menu. Fairly limited menu selections but lots of dessert selections!	No calorie or nutrition facts information on menu. Extremely decadent menu selections. Few light options. Low-carb options are a negative because they can deceive customers into thinking they're ordering healthy or low-cal meals (more on this below).	No calorie or nutrition facts information. Fairly limited menu.

Best Menu Choices							
Soups: •Chicken Broth with Lemongrass Soup Starters: •Tomato Salad or Mixed Greens with Endive, but always ask for dressing on the side so you can control how much you use. Just 2 level tablespoons of vinaigrette can provide 140 calories and 16 grams of fat. Burgers: •The Gardenburger could be a good choice if you omit the fried onion rings or french fries and ask for a side of steamed vegetables cooked without butter or oil — season them with black pepper at the table.	Any of them on the Eat Right menu. Because calorie information is provided, you will need a way of judging the calories against your calorie needs. Keep the basic formula in mind.*	They all look great, actually, but without the nutrition fact information it's hard to put in perspective — e.g., the Honey Ginger Dressing could be very light or very rich. All of the selections look nutrient-rich and lean. My recommendations: •Grilled Ginger Salmon •Market Fruit Salad as a dessert, with dressing on the side Because the	Same comments as for Hilton — they're all wonderful; you just need to know how to put these numbers in perspective for yourself.	•Seafood Chowder (if red, not cream variety) •Market Green Salad (dressing on the side) •Spiced Prawn and Avocado Salad, Oven Baked Crab and Mango Spring Rolls, Grilled Ahi Tuna, Chili Roasted Scallops and Prawns,	Difficult to say without complete nutrition facts information, but my picks would be as follows. Appetizers: •Cayman Style California Rolls •Fresh Fruit Mélange •Black Bean Soup (if not pork or meat based)	Difficult to say without complete nutrition facts information, but my picks would be as follows. Appetizers: •Seasonal Greens (dressing on the side) Entrées: •Grilled Chicken Sandwich — omit the fries and ask for a side of steamed vegetables cooked without butter or	Difficult to say without complete nutrition facts information, but my picks would be as follows. Appetizers: •Ensenada Cocktel Soups/Salads: •Local Baby Greens or Baby Spinach and Arugula — ask for light cheese and dressing on the side. Entrées: •Wild Salmon •Alaskan Halibut

InterContinental	Hilton	DoubleTree	Embassy Suites	Marriott	Westin	Sheraton	Kimpton
Entrées: • Grilled Ahi Tuna or Poached Salmon Fillet are good choices — but keep in mind that 3 to 4 ounces is considered a reasonable portion of seafood (about the size of a deck of cards or slightly larger). I doubt the portions are this small, so you could be doubling your protein portion here (and therefore your protein calories) if you eat more than 4 ounces. Also, no accompaniment is listed for these two (whereas the sole comes with new	Once you know your daily calorie needs, you can divide by 3 if you intend to eat three "square" meals a day to determine how many calories you have to spend at	nutrition fact information is available in the kitchen, I would guess that you can request it to help you make your decision.		Open Faced Smoked Salmon Tortilla, Grilled Chicken Spinach Wrap, and Open Faced Garden Sandwich all look to be great options, but it's difficult to say without complete nutrition facts information (the low-	• Cayman Conch Chowder (if not cream-based) *Salads/Sand-wiches:* • Cay-Mon Kay Salad, Organic Garden Salad, or Cayman Baby Greens Salad (all with dressing on side) • Blackened Grouper Sand-	oil — season them with black pepper at the table • Southwest Shrimp Wrap — ask for light cheese and guacamole on the side *Desserts:* If you want dessert, you should forgo the bun on the sandwich or the wrap, or order the Seasonal Greens and	• Tangerine Sautéed Shrimp (these all come with a starch, so if you plan to have dessert, ask to omit this). *Sides:* • Sautéed King Trumpet of Mushrooms and Warm Vegetable Slaw are likely prepared with a good deal of oil.

carb could be very high fat or the low-fat could be very high carb). Aside from these Fit for You selections, other good options include Wild Sockeye Salmon (without potatoes, unless you choose to spend your carbs here), Grilled Chicken Tagliatelle, and Grilled Butterflied

wich (sauce on the side) •Free Range Chicken Breast Sandwich (mayo on the side)—order sandwich with tropical fruit, not fries *Entrées:* •Top of the Catch (it doesn't say if it comes with anything such as potatoes)

ask for grilled chicken or shrimp on top—this will allow you to save some unspent carbs and fat on half a serving of dessert (or less, depending on how big they are).

which can up the calorie content quite a bit—if you plan to have dessert, ask for steamed vegetables, cooked without butter or oil, as a side.

potatoes), so ask about this to be sure—if it's served with a starch of some kind (potatoes, rice, etc.), avoid dessert or breads. Think about spending your carbs budget-style—if you spend on pasta or bread, you must save by skipping dessert.

breakfast, lunch, or dinner.

InterContinental	Hilton	DoubleTree	Embassy Suites	Marriott	Westin	Sheraton	Kimpton
				Breast of Chicken.	*Dessert:* If you're going to have dessert, limit the carbs and fat in your meal. A salad with grilled fish would help to balance the high fat and carb content of the Crème Brûlée, Rum		

Highest-Calorie Items on Menu	*Starters:* •California Farmhouse Cheese Platter *Burgers:* •Grilled Cheeseburger, with onion rings or fries (ugh!)	None! I read online that "menus were created by an exclu-	Can't say with cut complete facts on all items, but if they meet the Eat Right criteria, they are likely all	Same comments as for Hilton.	Where to begin? •Classic Caesar Salad •Classic Dry Garlic Ribs •Spicy	*Appetizers:* Where to begin? Nearly everything on this menu is rich, aside from what is listed

Cake, Key Lime Pie, or Napoleon –but do split it. Sorbets are low-fat, but they aren't generally low-calorie, so unless you love sorbet, splurge on half a rich dessert.

•Bruschetta (lots of oil and bread) •Quesadillas (too heavy

Nearly everything on this menu is rich, aside from what is listed above.

InterContinental	Hilton	DoubleTree	Embassy Suites	Marriott	Westin	Sheraton	Kimpton
Sandwiches: •Any of the club sandwiches, the Reuben, or the Egg Salad—just skip right over this section! *Pasta:* •Classic Lasagna, Lamb Ravioli *Entrées:* •The 12-ounce (yikes!) Sirloin with Pommes Frites, Filet Mignon with Short Ribs and Mashed Potatoes—you can just hear your arteries clogging here! My best guesstimate on the prix fixe dinner is approximately 2,500 calories, possibly 3,000 (because I don't know the portion sizes). This is far more calories than an average, moder-	sive team of Hilton Family of Hotels executive chefs who attended an intense five-day training course at the renowned Johnson & Wales University." The curriculum is focused around a nutritionally balanced diet, follow-ing the	reasonable calorie-wise.		Calamari (fried) •Any pasta dish •Veal Meatloaf, with mashed potatoes •Seafood Potpourri (cooked in butter) •Wiener Schnitzel—enough said •Cannelloni •Lamb, with mashed potatoes •Tenderloin, with pomme frites •The 12- or 14-ounce steaks! •BBQ Ribs	for an app) *Salads/Sandwiches:* •Caesar Club Sandwich (clubs usually mean lots of cheese and bacon) •Cuban Burger *Entrées:* •Cheese Ravioli •Caribbean Farfalle with Spicy Chicken (cream sauce)	above. I am not impressed with the low-carb options. Low-carb is a weight-loss fad—not a recognized recommended way of eating. There is no endorse-ment of a low-carb diet from the USDA, ADA, American Heart Association, American	

ately active adult needs all day and is about 2,000 to 2,500 over a recommended dinner calorie level. Also, the Dietary Guidelines recommend no more than one drink per day for women and two per day for men — one drink equals 5 ounces of wine.

guidelines set by the American Dietetic Association (ADA). As a spokesperson for the ADA, I can say that the meals all look balanced and nutrient-rich. I love that they include total calories, fat, protein, and carbs. No one of these

•Roast Beef Dip, with fries There are a lot of temptations here!

•Crab Cakes (heavy ingredients including wasabi mayo)
•Chicken Marsala (cream sauce)
Desserts:
•Banana Split (far too much ice cream and toppings to be reasonable, even if split)
•Sundae (if more than one scoop of ice cream).

Diabetes Association, or American Cancer Society. Why? Because it's not a balanced way of eating—in fact, the low-carb selections on this menu are some of the *least* healthy options (Buffalo Wings, New York Strip cooked in butter, burger with melted cheese,

InterContinental	Hilton	DoubleTree	Embassy Suites	Marriott	Westin	Sheraton	Kimpton
	is more important than another (sometimes you see only calories and fat and you miss the "big picture"—i.e., it's low-fat but is it super high carb?).					New York-Style Cheesecake—we're talking major saturated fat and cholesterol here! Heart disease is still a leading cause of death in the United States, and even thin people get heart disease. And the low-carb dishes could be very high in calories!	

General Nutrition/Fitness Notes:

1. Knowing the calorie and nutrition facts numbers is a huge plus. Low-fat, low-carb, vegetarian, or light meals aren't always low in calories, and the bottom line is that if you consume more calories than you burn, you will gain weight, regardless of what you're eating. However, in order to put calorie information into perspective, you need to know how many calories are right for you. Here's a quick and easy calculation.

*To maintain your *current* weight, the following formula can be used:

- 10 calories per pound of your body weight if you are sedentary or overweight
- 13 calories per pound of your body weight for low activity level (see below), or after the age of 55
- 15 calories per pound of your body weight for moderate activity (see below)
- 18 calories per pound of your body weight for strenuous activity (see below)Activity levels:

Activity levels:

- Low activity: No planned, regular daily physical activity; occasional weekend or recreational activities such as golf
- Moderate activity: Thirty to sixty minutes of physical activity like swimming, jogging, or fast walking most days of the week
- Strenuous activity: Sixty minutes or more of vigorous physical activity such as spinning class or racquetball, most days of the week

So a 165-pound adult with a low activity level needs about 2,145 calories to maintain his or her current weight.

2. Watch your alcohol intake. Alcohol can cause weight gain in three major ways. First, it's an appetite stimulant. Second, it causes you to lose your inhibitions—you may make menu choices you wouldn't make if you were sober! And finally, it's the mixers that'll get you. Sour mix, cream, cola, and the like, can add several hundred calories. If you do drink, try these tips:

- Stick with wine, a wine spritzer, light beer, or a mixed drink with a calorie-free mixer such as club soda, water, or diet soda—the lowest-calorie options.
- Drink a full glass of water between drinks—this is also to prevent dehydration and cut the risk of a hangover the next day, but it will also help reduce your total alcohol intake.

(Table footnote continued on next page.)

- Know the numbers. A 12-ounce light beer (standard bottle), a 5-ounce glass of wine (a little more than a mini-fruit cup), or a 1.5-ounce shot (shot glass) all provide about 100 calories and are all considered one drink. The 2005 Dietary Guidelines recommend a limit of one drink per day for women, two for men.

Even for professionals, it's difficult to guess what is healthy just by the menu, so I asked hotels to give us recipes for a few of their healthiest dishes from their menus. Based on that, here's a better picture of the real nutritional impact of the food offered at hotels.

APPENDIX A: NUTRITIONAL ANALYSIS OF HOTEL RECIPES

Hotel Chain	Recipe Name	Calories	Grams of Fat	Percentage of Calories from Fat	Grams of Saturated Fat	Percentage of Calories from Saturated Fat	Milligrams of Cholesterol	Grams of Fiber
DoubleTree	Kentucky Onion Ribeye	460	12	23.48%	4.5	8.80%	110	8
DoubleTree	Margo Oatmeal	270	8	26.67%	1.5	5%	5	4
DoubleTree	Parmesan Frittata served with Sweet Potato and Poblano Chili Hash	410	9	19.76%	2.5	5.49%	140	11
DoubleTree	Sautéed Salmon	300	13	39%	2.5	7.5%	70	3
Embassy Suites	Cold Cucumber Dill Soup	130	0	0%	0	0%	5	1
Embassy Suites	Grilled Free-Range Chicken	270	6	20%	1.5	5%	20	10
Embassy Suites	Grilled Tortilla Pizza	290	12	37.24%	3.5	10.86%	5	7
Embassy Suites	Pepper Tuna with Cucumber Fennel Salad	410	22	48.29%	4	8.78%	55	4
Four Seasons*	Four Seasons Multi-Grain Pancakes with Seasonal Fruit Compote	491	16.28	29.85%	1.91	3.5%	4.9	7.29
Four Seasons*	Grilled Pineapple, Hearts of Palm, Asparagus & Baby Greens Salad	177	0.93	4.7%	0.18	0.91%	0	5.48
Four Seasons*	Grilled Swordfish with Rice Beans, Artichokes, Tomato-Fennel Stew, Olive Caper Relish	612	24.83	36.48%	5.39	7.92%	84.37	18.45

APPENDIX A: NUTRITIONAL ANALYSIS OF HOTEL RECIPES (Continued)

Hotel Chain	Recipe Name	Calories	Grams of Fat	Percentage of Calories from Fat	Grams of Saturated Fat	Percentage of Calories from Saturated Fat	Milligrams of Cholesterol	Grams of Fiber
Four Seasons*	Vegetarian Bento Box	255	7.94	27.99%	1.22	4.29%	4.18	7.92
Hilton	Chilled Tarragon Chicken and Arugula Salad	230	7	27.39%	3	11.74%	180	2
Hilton	Egg White Frittata Wrap	350	10	25.71%	2	5.14%	0	8
Hilton	Fried Zucchini Quesadilla	390	25	57.69%	10	23.08%	45	3
Hilton	Grilled Ginger Salmon	240	10	37.5%	1.5	5.63%	20	5
Kimpton*	Basic Fruit Paletta	86	0.29	3%	0.03	0.34%	0	0.27
Kimpton*	Chipotle Grilled Chicken with Avocado Salsa	711	42.38	53.65%	10.3	13.04%	197.34	4.42
Kimpton*	Jsix Corn and Poblano Soup	145	6.52	40.39%	1.68	10.38%	5.82	3.24
Kimpton*	Roasted Chicken with Caramelized Garlic and Sage served over Lemon Risotto	904	30.99	30.85%	9.32	9.28%	93.83	1.43
Kimpton*	Seared Shrimp with Tangerine, Cilantro, and Pasilla Chile	201	7.55	33.88%	2.58	11.57%	187.73	1.14
Kimpton*	Truffle Salt Salmon and Four-Onion Patina	585	30.22	46.46%	10.27	15.79%	136.6	2.57
Marriott	Broiled Pacific Salmon	617	19	27.71%	7	10.21%	286	4
Marriott	Pan-Seared Halibut	196	1	4.59%	0	0%	11	1
Radisson*	Pan-Seared Atlantic Salmon with Warm Artichoke and Tomato Salad with Lemon Dressing	561	23.14	37.12%	3.44	5.53%	125.6	16.56

Ritz*	Braised Caesar Salad	439	39.83	81.74%	11.47	23.54%	32.24	2.53
Ritz*	Maine Lobster Shabu-Shabu	737	3.28	4.01%	0.53	0.65%	212.4	10.37
Ritz*	Salmon Tartare with Meyer Lemon and Avocado	418	26.88	57.9%	5.13	11.05%	99.28	4.64
Sheraton*	California Cobb Salad	95	65.65	62.1%	16.77	13.85%	381.3	9.67
Sheraton*	Cay-mon Kay Salad	761	51.61	61.04%	10.22	12.09%	136.41	6.28
Sheraton*	Chicken Breast Salad	426	28.87	60.97%	4.73	9.99%	74.04	2.6
Sheraton*	Miso Salmon	635	22.88	32.43%	4.95	7.02%	130.77	11.07
Sheraton*	Seasonal Greens Salad	84	6.47	69.45%	0.5	5.4%	2.37	2.22
Westin*	Angel Hair Pasta with Sautéed Chicken	638	23.43	33.03%	4.3	6.07%	57.73	5.68
Westin*	Poached Seabass served with Guava, Leek, and Onion Chiffonade, Sautéed Spinach, and Petit Vegetables	353	9.62	24.55%	1.76	4.5%	105.86	5.26
Westin*	Salmon and Tuna Ceviche with Leche de Tigre and Crispy Marikitas	385	19.64	45.85%	11.78	27.51%	88.2	2.5
Westin*	Seared Tuna Salad	720	46.03	57.54%	10.78	13.48%	132.13	11.19
Wyndham*	Grilled Salmon with Warm Potato and Spinach Salad	632	37.67	53.64%	11.78	16.78%	173.51	3.13
Wyndham*	Roasted Chicken Breast Saltimbocca	603	31.13	46.44%	7.11	10.61%	118.19	5.83

*Nutrition information was estimated from recipes provided by hotel chains.

And just about the time you were starting to feel pretty good about the healthy intentions of hotel menus, a report from the Physicians Committee for Responsible Medicine weighed in (so to speak) on this issue. The PCRM nutrition professionals likewise asked hotel chains to provide recipes for their "healthiest" menu items. DoubleTree, Embassy Suites, Hilton, and Marriott recipes contained a nutritional analysis. That information was used, and the percentages of calories from fat and saturated fat were calculated. Their results were not heartening: The PCRM determined that many meal options described as promoting health or fitness are actually surprisingly high in fat and cholesterol, which can contribute to heart disease and diabetes.

Hilton, DoubleTree, and Embassy Suites

The PCRM applauded Hilton for providing nutrient information on their Eat Right menu. Among the PCRM's best choices are the vegetarian items, such as Mango Oatmeal and Scrambled Tofu with Potato at breakfast and the Roasted Vegetable and Sun-Dried Hummus Wrap at lunch and dinner. But these hotels also serve some far less healthful options. Hilton, for example, features such high-fat, high-cholesterol offerings as Hearty Braised Beef Stew and Roast Lamb Loin.

InterContinental

Most menus the PCRM reviewed from InterContinental do not make an effort to point out any healthy items that might be available. However, a few of the menus marked some items with a heart symbol, which is typically used to denote foods with reduced calories, cholesterol, fat, and sodium. The best of these options are the Grilled Stuffed Eggplant, the Eastern Mediterranean Wrap, the Tofu Napoleon with Vegetables, and the Fresh Seasonal Berries for dessert. Unfortunately, many items marked with this heart symbol (such as the New Yorker Salad, which includes eggs and bacon among its ingredients) contained too many animal products to actually be considered healthy.

Marriott

Some of Marriott's options deserve their healthy label—White Bean and Arugula Salad, Vegetable Stir-Fry, and Whole Wheat Penne Pasta with Tomato Basil Sauce, for example. However, many items in this line contain fatty meat and cheese and are likely to raise cholesterol levels, not lower them. Another problem with Marriott's "Fit for You" menu is that some items are marked as being "carb-conscious" or "low-carb." These include the Char-Grilled 12-Ounce New York Steak (served with fried onion rings) and the Cobb Salad, which contains chicken, bacon, eggs, blue cheese, and cheddar cheese. These items are fad-conscious, not health-conscious. Carbohydrate-restricted, high-protein diets are associated with health risks ranging from constipation, headache, and bad breath to more significant problems such as cholesterol elevation and calcium loss.

Ritz-Carlton

The children's menu was reviewed here. According to the PCRM, although some of the menu options are more healthful than those found on typical children's menus, several items (such as the Satay Beef and the Ground Beef Burger) are still heavy on the fatty meats and cheeses. Better choices include "Ants on the Lake" (peanut butter, raisins, and celery), Herb Roasted New Potato Wedges instead of the standard french fries, and fresh fruit with sorbet for dessert. One menu even offers edamame (green soybeans) as an appetizer for kids. These are laudable choices, given the increasing obesity problem among America's children.

Westin

Some Westin hotel menus include items marked as healthy, though the terminology varies depending on the hotel (terms include "Smart Dining," "Spa Cuisine—Westin Smart Dining," "Healthy Heart Options," "Westin Smart One Dining," and "Health Smart Menu Suggestions"). But many items marked as healthy actually contain high-fat and high-cholesterol ingredients. Among these unhealthful choices are the Honey Glazed Duck Breast and the Certified Angus Beef Grilled Teriyaki Flat Iron Steak. Items lowest in fat and cholesterol are the vegetarian choices, such as the Heirloom Tomato and Summer Melon Salad, the Veggie Burger, and the Vegetarian Penne Pasta.

Conclusion

At least six major hotel chains (Kimpton, Hyatt, Sheraton, Wyndham, Four Seasons, and Radisson) are not making any apparent attempt to offer healthier meals. Other hotels are making an effort, but it is still up to the health-conscious diner to pick and choose carefully, even among the supposedly healthful offerings.

The bottom line: Eater beware. Even the most well-intentioned hotel menus can be traps. Once again, it's a matter of basic common sense, portion control, and . . . timing.

Basic common sense tells us that if we're traveling, even with fast-food choices, we should choose a salad. Not necessarily so. The PCRM analyzed the salad choices at fast-food restaurants, and the results were shocking. McDonald's Bacon Ranch Salad with Crispy Chicken has *more* fat and calories and just as much cholesterol as a Big Mac. And the Chef Salad at Au Bon Pain is loaded with more than 1,300 milligrams of sodium. So, although in general it's smart to choose a salad over a burger, be sure to read the fine print.

Then there's portion control. Heidi Skolnik taught me to fight my conditioning, and when ordering from hotel or restaurant menus, order two appetizers but no entrée, or one entrée and no appetizers, and I'd be better off. She was right.

Finally, there's timing. And this is the toughest part, especially for business travelers on the road. Just about every nutritionist will recommend that you eat dinner before 8 P.M. That's virtually impossible if you're out of town and entertaining clients or friends. But there's a way around this. If your dinner reservations are for after 8 P.M. no points will be deducted from your final score for ordering a simple salad as your entrée. And remember my pilot friend's advice about the salad dressing? Again, order it on the side, and then . . . stick a fork in it, (use the fork to apply the dressing). Another point about timing. According to many researchers, when you're eating, you really become full about ten minutes before it actually registers in your brain. So, what I have learned to do is stop eating when I'm about three-quarters finished with my food. It works.

The same principles apply when you are eating outside the hotel, of course, but in this case, the rules are even tougher and the challenges greater. Assuming you'll be staying at a hotel for three nights, the odds are excellent that you'll eat inside the hotel on only one of those three nights. And for many travelers, the real problem with eating out happens when they leave the hotel for meals.

For example, I have always been a big fan of Asian cuisine when I travel. And, as I've discovered, that's a major nutrition and calorie disaster. In 1993, the Center for Science in the Public Interest looked at Chinese restaurant meals, and the results were shocking. If you want calories, fat, and sodium in supersized amounts, then Chinese food is one-stop shopping. The CSPI research revealed that a single entrée of Kung Pao Chicken and Rice—which sounds harmless enough—contained 1,600 calories, 76 grams of fat, and 2,600 milligrams of sodium.

The CSPI also targeted salad dressings and meat as two other major sources of fat at major city restaurants. Now I'm not suggesting that you don't eat meat—I'm as far away from a vegan as you could possibly get, and I love salad dressing. Again, it's a matter of what time you eat and portion control—a filet mignon is a better choice than a full ribeye—and, of course, how you eat—for example, the fork finesse when it comes to salad dressing.

But eating—how much, what, and when—is just part of the hotel equation when it comes to the traveler's diet. The next part, perhaps the hardest, is . . . exercise. No, I take that back. Delete the word "perhaps." Exercise *is* the hardest. And believe me, I'm just *writing* about this, and I feel the pain . . .

CHAPTER 6

Sweat Equity

I have never taken any exercise
except sleeping and resting.

—*Mark Twain*

I don't care what anyone else tells you about exercise. If they say they love to do it, they're lying. If they insist it's fun, they are delusional. And if they can't wait to get up in the morning to run to the gym, then I just don't trust these people.

To me, exercise has always been nothing less, and nothing more, than doing penance for my past sins—of overeating, not eating right, and simply not taking care of myself at home and especially on the road. Of course, if I had a simpler, more manageable, nine-to-five structure to my days, I'd only have somewhat less of an excuse not to exercise, and not to write this book. The point is—at least to me—that exercise has always been a punishment, not a goal. And that's why I never looked forward to it. Until now.

Heidi Skolnik said it best when she said my goal was to provide structure in my unstructured world of travel. And this should be your goal as well.

So how do you incorporate regular exercise into that unstructured environment? This was my biggest challenge, and it remains my biggest challenge. The good news is that I was able to figure it out. And when you consider my travel schedule, if I can do that, anyone can.

Welcome to my brave new world of . . . sweat equity.

I started my exercise program in New York—appropriately, at a hotel. Trainer Annette Lang and I began using the gym/health club at the New York Sheraton, on West 53rd Street. And we averaged two days a week there. But that wasn't enough. The other two days a week would have to happen on the road.

This was a challenge for both of us. Annette would have to work hard to get me up to speed on my routines, and I would have to work harder to maintain those levels on the road. She would be with me at each session at the hotel gym. But I'd have to exercise greater discipline and determination on the road.

Annette kept a detailed diary of my workouts, tracking not only my successes but also my failures (I told you this wasn't easy . . .). Here are some of her initial diary entries:

"Peter knows he is deconditioned, and this will be tough for him."
"I planned a circuit workout so that he gets cardio and full body; goal is to do two to three circuits, two to three times each week."

Annette and I also talked about my being more active in general—walking more, taking stairs instead of escalators at the airport, and taking advantage of activities possible in cities where I travel.

While Annette designed a workout specifically for me, the blueprint will work for many a couch potato.

- Full-body routine to be done at least two to three times per week
  —The objective is to get as much movement as possible. Since Peter is deconditioned, this means his exercise intensity will be low to moderate as tolerable for the first six to eight weeks.
  —Strength training will be done at moderate intensity, that is twelve to fifteen reps with adequate resistance to achieve fatigue but not failure. He has not exercised in a long time, so we need to take the time to get all the joints and stabilizer muscles stronger so we avoid injuries as he is exercising more.
  —Full-body routines will include these exercises and movements:
  Lower body: Modified dead lifts, bridges, standing positions while doing upper-body exercises
  Upper body: Pulling exercises (rows, pulldowns, pullovers) Pushing exercises (pushups, chest presses)

Core training: Stability postures in different positions
Stretching: Peter doesn't seem to need

Range of motion is OK.

Overall strength is my concern more than stretching.

Program will change according to functional variables:

Changing angles

Moving along all three planes

—Peter does not feel comfortable doing lunges and squats because of an ACL repair done years ago. He reports feeling pressure in the area. Program will start with leg press options, or modified dead lifts and bridges, until he becomes more fit and can handle the weight on the knee. For bridges, lie on the floor with knees bent and feet on the floor, lift up hips; works glutes and hamstrings.

- Focus is on cables, machines, and free weights.
  —He needs variety just in case the hotel has only one type.

- Cardio intervals will be included.
  —Will determine precise parameters at our first training session July 28, but most likely three intervals at moderate intensity for two to four minutes each, to start.

- Workout will be set up in a circuit fashion, for example, doing a series of different exercises for the entire body and then doing another round of either the same exercises or different ones. The advantage is that even if you go through only one round or circuit, you are addressing the entire body.

- This is an important consideration when people are traveling. They either get out of their original plan, or don't plan ahead enough, or think that if they do a little bit, then it won't be good enough. Doing a circuit workout gets you going the first round, and then many times that is enough to get yourself motivated to do more and to be more active and stick to your eating habits the rest of the day.

Our first workout together lasted a total of eighteen minutes, and included the following:

Treadmill	3.0 mph	7% incline, 5 minutes
Lat pulldown	80 pounds	15 reps
Leg curl	40 pounds	Right knee discomfort after 9 reps
Bridge on stability ball	15 reps with Annette holding ball	
Reverse crunch	8 reps	
Reverse fly on combo/ chest machine	40 pounds	
Straight-arm pulldown cable	70 pounds	
Shoulder press	15 pounds	15 reps—challenging
Lateral stability hold on knees	5 seconds	three times
Bridge again		
Reverse crunch again		
Lateral hold again		

Annette started me with a lot of machine choices, since many health clubs do not have as many free weights. And sitting helped me learn form and still get some stability because my legs were under the support pad.

Here are Annette's notes from the first session:

• *Leg curl:* In case he only has machines on the road as a choice; we needed to get and keep his hamstrings and glutes strong to help the knee get stronger as well.

- *Bridge on the ball:* I held the ball to make it easier to stabilize; need to get those glutes stronger! Also great for the core.

- *Reverse crunch:* Decided on these as opposed to traditional ones, since those put a lot of stress on the upper middle back/upper traps. These muscles are traditionally "tight"; full of tension when the rest of the body/core, relative to itself, needs to get stronger. So the reverse crunches make Peter get in touch with the deep ab stabilizers. He said he really feels them, too. Trying to coordinate his breathing; to initiate the movement with breathing.

- *Reverse fly on machine:* Machine just in case that is the only choice he has. Also, when working the upper middle back and back of the shoulders, it is very easy to compensate when the body is not strong enough from the inside out and begin to shrug the shoulders and strain the neck.

- *Straight-arm pulldown with cable:* This is great because you have to stand while doing the exercise. You have to hold yourself still while doing the exercise. It also works your triceps as well as your lats.

- *Shoulder press:* Working the shoulders and arms while standing. This is important for real-life activities like putting your luggage into the overhead bin in the airplane!

- *Lateral stability hold on knees:* This is an example of an exercise that challenges your relative strength. Relative strength means how strong you are relative to your weight or mass. This is why the boot camp workouts became more popular the last several years, because people wanted to be stronger at moving their own bodies! This exercise is really good to help stabilize the spine, the SI (sacroiliac) joint, which is crucial for low back health, and the core, which is the whole midsection of the body.

Before our first workout, Annette also took basic measurements. And, not surprising, it was embarrassing to see those numbers:

Chest	50.25 inches
Right arm	15.25 inches
Left arm	15 inches
Smallest part of waist	51 inches
Hips	48.75 inches

Our next workout was four days later. And, as I'd come to expect, Annette kept score:

Elliptical Life Fitness Manual Level 3	50 rpm	5 minutes
Straight-arm pulldown	70-pound cable	
Band walking	15 feet	two times back and forth
Hold position, biceps curl	15-pound dumbbells	15 reps
Cable core rotation, standing	3 plates	
Cable chest fly, standing	2 plates	
Dead lift	15-pound dumbbells	needs better form
Shoulder press	15-pound dumbbells	15 reps
Treadmill	3 mph	7% incline, 5 minutes
Lat pulldown	80 pounds	12 reps—harder today after one circuit

Leg curl	40 pounds	15 reps—good
Reverse fly, machine	40 pounds	
Single-arm cable row with opposite leg in front	3 plates	hard
Pushup, on knees	10 reps	
Reverse crunch	15 reps	really feels them
Ball bridge	15 reps	needs more lift
Lateral hold, on knees	5 seconds	3 times
Reverse crunch	15 reps	
Elliptical	same as before	
Reverse fly, cable	80 pounds	standing
Overhead press	15 pounds	15 reps
Dead lift again	better	
Core rotation again		
Hip bridge on ball again		
Hamstring stretch	right side tighter	
Pec stretch, leaning against ball		

I was wasted after this session, but it felt so much better. And—we had gone from eighteen minutes to a full hour.

Here are Annette's comments on the session:

- *Elliptical:* Peter liked the movement pattern, and it's good because it gets the upper body moving at the same time.

- *Band walking:* (Peter called this one the "hostage walk.") I gave Peter the band; it's a simple band that you put around your thighs, stand with some tension in the band, then walk side to side. It is to work the outer hips and glutes. The outer hips are vital to knee health and to get those glutes working again! I told him how knee problems are many times caused by foot/ankle and/or hip problems. So he walked back and

forth about 15 feet, twice. Then he stood there and did biceps curls with dumbbells.

- *Biceps curl:* Not a vital exercise, but you gotta have your arms
look good! By doing this with the band around the thighs, he
got some great interconnection—outer hip and upper body
exercise, with the goal again being to work as much as possible with each exercise eventually.

- *Standing cable core rotation:* Great to work the core, and to
teach the body to work together. You pull the cable from the
left, turning your whole body to the right. Remember to exhale as you start the movement.

- *Cable chest fly:* Working the muscles in the front, but while
standing, to challenge the core muscles, and overall balance
and stability. While standing in between the cable columns,
you pull from either side, as if putting your arms around a big
tree. You keep the elbows soft, and exhale as you pull. You
can put one foot in front of the other for more stability.

- *Dead lift:* With dumbbells. We need to work the glutes and
hamstrings, without a lot of knee bending because of that
right knee. Dead lifts are great for the low back, too. He
needs to keep working on the form, keeping the natural
curves in the low back, as he hinges forward from the hips.

- *Row with cable, standing:* Pull cable with right arm while
standing with left leg in front of the right. The body's muscles attach in diagonal lines, so the right lats work well with
the left butt muscles. Standing in this position addresses this
relationship.

- *Hamstring stretch:* Just want to do moderate static stretch to
help him feel good, and to make sure the range of motion is

close to the same with the right and left leg. Right side was tighter than the left, and I know it makes him feel uncomfortable when doing this with the right side.

- *Pec stretch:* Sitting on the floor, leaning against the stability ball, with his head on a towel to maintain neutral spine. I hold his elbows, as he is putting his hand behind his head. He loved this; besides a nice stretch in the anterior muscles, this is great against the stability ball to achieve thoracic extension.

We were starting to get into a groove. And I was beginning to anticipate each new exercise in sequence, so I knew where I was in the circuit. This was important to me because my new goal—at each session—was not to do any more exercises or increase my reps. It was just . . . to finish it!

And as we exercised more, Annette shared with me her philosophy. "There are no magic exercises," she said. "You just need to get your body moving more. This is not about six-pack abs, it's about simply getting in shape and staying in shape."

Annette isn't a fitness nut, but she is definitely a fitness professional. "A lot of us get into this field because of what happened to them and/or their family, like losing a bunch of weight, or having heart disease in the family, she explained. "I remember being a kid and just being happy with myself, and noticing how unhappy a lot of people are, with the work, their spouse, themselves, etc. I also noticed that staying active helped my self-image and self-esteem and made me feel good, and motivated me in other endeavors of my life. So I thought if I could help others get more active, it might spur them on to make other positive changes in their lives. So my whole career has been focusing on that—personal training, and also teaching personal trainers. My master's degree in health education is more important than any exercise science class I took, because if someone doesn't want to change, I can't begin to help them."

Ten days after our first workout, I was down another 3 pounds. And from that point on, I began to drop between a pound and a pound-and-a-half a week.

I felt the difference. I became out of breath less quickly. I felt muscles forming, especially the abs, which was encouraging. As I improved, Annette also increased the number of reps—twelve push-ups instead of ten—and added exercises, like rotations, where I start out on my back with legs up and knees bent, then rotate six times to each side.

Here is my new routine:

- Started with things he can do on his own as reinforcement.

Stability ball bridge	15 reps	I held the ball less than last time
Reverse crunch	12 instead of 10	
Lateral hold	8 seconds each side	that looked easier
Pushup	12 instead of 10	

- Added rotations—lying on back with legs up and knees bent, rotate six times to each side.

- Same round again; we changed the lateral holds to where his legs were in a straight line, since it seemed like he could do it: five seconds each side.

- Two sets of the following:

Lat pulldown	80 pounds	15 reps
Leg curl	40 pounds	15 reps—better later, when his knee is warmer
Dead lift	15 pounds	15 reps—form is better
Biceps curl, overhead press	15 pounds	difficult but did 12 reps; told him to relax, which was better
Cable straight-arm pulldown	70 pounds	still needs to keep those shoulders down and back

Cable core rotation	3 plates	he really feels these

- One set of the following:

Chest press with dumbbells instead of cable	15 pounds	difficult for 12 reps
Reverse fly, machine	40 pounds	
Single-arm row with cable	3 plates	
Elliptical, on his own	15 minutes	

Our next workout was not a great one. My schedule changed. I couldn't make the appointments. I was at the same weight as the week before. I had not done enough exercise on my own, and I had slipped in the eating department as well. I had eaten one too many bagels in the *Today* show greenroom. It was time for a lecture from Annette. From her notes:

Peter needs to come to grips with what needs to be done. I am telling him, and also asking him to tell me . . .

What is it that enticed him to travel as much as he does in the first place—besides the fact that it is a huge, successful business now? Traveling by its sheer definition encompasses a sense of movement and being mobile and active. Can't he build that into it and uncover a whole other purpose to his shows and programs? Showing he can do this on the road is not just about walking on the treadmill in the gym. What is it going to take for P. to change his attitude? Does he want to get these results and, more important, live a different lifestyle than he has been, because what I saw yesterday in the gym made me think the answer is that he is not sure yet.

He asked about how many calories I think he is burning during one workout, and research has shown that an average circuit workout like what we are doing burns about 200 to 300 calories or so. The point of the workout is to not lose muscle because of the dieting, and help his health and fitness level. But one workout each week is not going to get the results we need if he does as little on his own as he has the last two weeks.

I was surprised these workouts that required such energy expenditure burned so few calories! This was not encouraging. No wonder people don't exercise. But I persevered because I saw no way around it.

Elliptical	Level 3	5 minutes
Cable straight-arm pulldown	7 plates	15 reps seemed difficult
Cable full-body rotation	3 plates	15 reps
Band walking, side to side, then holding position and biceps curl, overhead press	15 pounds	12 reps— difficult today
Leg curl	4 plates	15 reps
Single-arm row on cable	3 plates	
Treadmill	3 mph	7% incline, 5 minutes; had to hold on several times for a total of about 1 minute; I don't like this because it screws up your gait.
Pushup	did 12 on toes	
Reverse crunch	18 reps, which is a few more	
Side hold	can't do with straight legs yet; did 10-second holds with knees bent	

Bridge with lower body on ball		
Did not do the rotations we introduced last week		
Lat pulldown	80 pounds	much better form; needs to slow down
Dead lift	15 pounds	15 reps
Reverse fly on cable	4 plates	good form
Biceps curls, overhead press	15 pounds	15 reps—much better form
Reverse fly, machine	3 plates	15 reps, and then that was it

I only had a year to lose 60 pounds, and I couldn't afford to backslide. I was determined to ramp it up. And our next workout a few days later reflected that.

From Annette's notes:

- He said he wanted to work harder, so we did intervals on the cardio. Plus two workouts in a row (today and tomorrow); I had to make them somewhat different.

- Interval of 10 minutes alternated between 7 and 10 percent incline and 3 mph; this circuit two times.

Leg press, squat press machine	35 pounds each side	liked it; good for legs
Lat pulldown	80 pounds	much better form
Pushup	12 reps	better
Reverse crunch	15 reps	
Side planks	10 seconds	got into straighter line but still on knees
Elliptical interval	8 to 10 or so; 1:1 minute	took time to get proper numbers

- This circuit twice:

Leg curl	4 plates	too easy
Cable straight-arm pulldown	7 plates	
Same cable, rear delts		
Overhead press	15 pounds	15 reps, then 12
Biceps curls	15 pounds	15, then 12 reps
Ball bridges	15 reps	I am holding the ball a little less than when we started. His balance will be challenged until we get that core stronger so I don't want to dwell on it too much.
Rotation	8 times each side	
Elliptical	6 minutes	

- Much better workout!

And the next workout got even better. . . . Here are Annette's notes:

- We did an interval/circuit right by the elliptical.

- Alternated this 2.5 times: elliptical; exercises; elliptical; exercises; elliptical.

- Elliptical for six minutes, six to seven level alternates; 1:1 minute intervals.

- Walking pushups, 15, 10: change angle from which and to which you move, to make the joints work harder in different positions; good for variety and for joint stability/integrity.

- Seated rotations with 10 pounds; eight each side; he really felt this in his midsection. This exercise is great for the core. You are rotating, which is something we didn't do in fitness for way too long, and you get the muscles all around the midsection. Considering the time he spends sitting in an airplane, this one will help his back.

- Prone holds; six seconds—very difficult; on knees; his relative strength is poor; "your body against gravity" is what I was telling him! He starts shaking pretty quickly, which is a sign of fatigue. Your whole body is working isometrically to hold still against gravity, which is not easy.

This circuit twice:

- Hip extension on slant board with 10 pounds in front—much better form than when doing dead lifts; really felt them. Lean on the slant board; keeping natural curve in low back, lean forward from hip as far as possible without losing curve in low back; come back up; works glutes and hamstrings.

- Single-arm rows with 15-pound dumbbell. He looks a little sloppy on this one still; it's just a matter of time until his core gets stronger and he is in more control of his own body!

- Hammer strength chest press, 35 pounds each side. He likes this one, and I am sure it has something to do with the fact that he gets to sit down and be supported by the machine, which is OK with me at this point!

- Pullovers on bench with 15-pound dumbbell; hard. This exercise targets the lats, but you also get the abs because they have to keep you still as your arms go overhead.

- Leg press, 35 pounds each side. He likes this one, and I am glad because we need to get that lower body better.

Two days later, the next workout:

Elliptical intervals	Level 8 to 10	total 10 minutes
Two exercises	3 reps each	
Leg press	35 then 45 pounds each side	
Pushup	12 to 15 reps	
Hip extension	10-pound weight	
Lat pulldown	80 pounds	
Single-arm biceps curl, overhead press	15 pounds	

- Felt low back discomfort on right side; went back to elliptical.

I returned the next morning:

Elliptical	Level 7, steady pace	8 minutes
3 sets with short rest		
Hammer strength chest press	25-, 35-, 40-pound	
Leg curl	4.5, 5, 15 reps	
Barbell rows	20 pounds each side	
Single-arm row	25, 30 pounds	
Ball bridge		
Seated rotation	10 pounds	
Supine hold	8 seconds	
Lateral hold	8 seconds	
Prone hold	8 seconds	

Elliptical	6 minutes	increased the rpms to 60 to 70; he was wasted

- He said he liked the workout, possibly because he liked the short recovery in between sets, but he did work hard, too!

- He definitely is doing better with the workouts. He took several meetings to become familiar with some movement patterns, and because he does not come from a gym background as far as exercise programs, I started putting him on more machines to make it easier.

When I started, I liked the treadmill and dreaded the elliptical machine because it looked like a StairMaster, which I hated. But soon, it was just the opposite. Annette started me on intervals, going from Level 8 to Level 10, and then back again. A minute on, and a minute at two higher levels. And then, between Levels 10 and 12. And then, once I got going beyond the five- or six-minute mark, it was easy to hit Level 10; once beyond 14, I could make twenty minutes; and once I hit 24, there was no way I wasn't going to make it to thirty minutes. And now I often do this at Level 13 all the way.

One reason I like the elliptical more than the treadmill is that I tire more easily on the treadmill. Reason: I expend more energy on the treadmill! (What a surprise.) The elliptical pedals move with me, which lessens the impact, whereas on the treadmill, I have to lift and land on my legs, and that's harder on the muscles. Still, I'd pick the elliptical over the treadmill any day.

Regardless, the weight kept dropping. Four months into the workout regime, and I had lost almost 22 pounds. It was beginning to show. Friends and coworkers were starting to give me compliments, and that positive reinforcement was—and continues to be—a great motivator.

Although I still hadn't changed all my bad patterns—I was not eating proper breakfasts, for example—I was doing something I never thought I'd do: I kicked the Diet Pepsi habit. I went from twenty-two cans a day (I never actually finished one), down to four, then to two, and then, after a stern lecture by my friend and chef Jimmy Boyce, down to . . . none.

And here's the interesting part (of course, I didn't know it at the time): People who drink diet sodas don't lose weight—in fact, they *gain* weight. And for addicted Diet Pepsi freaks like me—people who thought drinking diet soda on the road would somehow counterbalance all the other bad things—it was nothing short of a revelation.

Gain weight by drinking diet soda? That's the finding, after eight years of research at the University of Texas Science Center in San Antonio. "What didn't surprise us was that total soft drink use was linked to overweight and obesity," said one of the researchers. "What was surprising was when we looked at people only drinking diet soft drinks, their risk of obesity was even higher."

How could that be? The University of Texas team studied about 1,550 people ranging in age from twenty-four to sixty-two. For those who consumed more than two regular cans of soft drink a day, the risk of becoming overweight was 47.2 percent. No surprises there. But then the researchers analyzed the diet soda drinkers, and the numbers were shocking: For those who were drinking more than two cans a day, the risk of becoming overweight was 57.1 percent!

No, diet soda does *not* cause obesity. Instead, the research indicated that there is something linked to drinking diet soda that is also linked to obesity. Perhaps the best explanation for these numbers is not the diet soda that's consumed, but what is on your plate.

Specifically, and simply, it's this: People who drink diet soda think that consuming diet drinks means they're maintaining the diet, and that they then somehow have permission to eat . . . well, crap. In fact, it may also mean that we actually crave *more* calories when we drink diet soda. In another study, when laboratory rats were fed artificial sweeteners, they ate more than the rats fed real sugar!

But there's another effect as well.

In the first week after I stopped the Diet Pepsi, I found myself in bed every night at 8 P.M. Explanation: I was literally coming down from my caffeine habit. And then, about a week later, I stabilized back to my old routine.

I replaced the Diet Pepsi with water. I began with the equation whereby I would drink—in ounces—one-half of the pounds I weighed. Starting at 284 pounds, that meant about 140 ounces of water a day. By the end of the summer, I was down to about 261 pounds, and that meant about 130 ounces of water a day. It became an effective tool in my weight-loss program.

Indeed, I did make a lot more visits to the bathroom—a *lot* more—but it was worth it on so many other levels. The increase in water consumption meant a great improvement in my metabolism, and at the same time, I found myself no longer munching between meals. I wasn't hungry at weird hours. And perhaps the most surprising (and pleasant) discovery: Two 8-ounce bottles of water late at night meant absolutely no midnight snacking!

I knew something about kidney function and water. But then I learned about the relationship between water, liver function, and the metabolism of fats. The liver is crucial in converting and utilizing fat for energy. And if my liver is functioning well, then I have a better chance of burning that extra fat.

Then there are the basics to consider. My body, your body—everyone's body—needs about 2 liters of water a day just to function. If you exercise, add another 750 milliliters for every hour you work out. But the water is also essential as a mechanism to help weight loss. At one research center in Berlin, scientists studied the caloric intake and energy expenditure of men and women who drank two glasses of water a day. Within ten minutes of drinking water, their metabolic rate increased by a staggering 30 percent. And that's with just two glasses of water!

In men, the increased metabolism was manifested by fat breakdown (and with women, both fat and carbohydrate breakdown). But the most significant finding was that the researchers estimated that drinking just 1.5 liters of water a day could, over the course of a year, result in a weight loss of approximately 5 pounds.

And I was drinking a lot more than that.

Put in proper perspective, water isn't the only answer, but it certainly became part of my total answer to the overall weight-loss challenge.

In the meantime, my workouts in New York continued to increase in both frequency and intensity:

Elliptical	Level 8	6 minutes
Flat chest press	25-pound dumbbells	15 reps
Lat pulldown	80 pounds, overhand grip	15 reps
Scaption	10-pound dumbbells, standing	15 reps
Leg press	45-pound plate on each side	15 reps
Treadmill	3.2 mph	5% incline, 6 minutes
Chest fly, Cybex machine	60 pounds	15 reps
Single-arm row	25-pound dumbbell, one arm/leg on bench for support	15 reps
Rear delts, Cybex machine	40 pounds	15 reps
Leg curl	40 pounds	15 reps

Elliptical	Level 8	6 minutes
Incline chest press	25-pound dumbbells	15 reps
Lat pulldown, underhand grip	80 pounds	15 reps
Curl and press, standing	15-pound dumbbells	15 reps
Leg extension	60 pounds	15 reps
Treadmill	3.2 mph	5% incline, 6 minutes
Bridge	supine on floor, knees bent, soles of feet on stability ball	15 reps
Reverse crunch	knees bent on stability ball, knees to chest lifting ball/hips off floor	15 reps
Crunch	knees bent on stability ball, alternating diagonal sit-ups	20 reps
Bicycle sit-up	knees bent, feet on floor, alternating, opposite elbow to knee	20 reps

By September 26, 2005, just a few months after starting, my weight dipped below 260, down to 258—26 pounds lighter than when I began. I was starting to eat fruit for breakfast. No more bagels.

This was—and remains—so tough for me. But I now had the motivation. I could see the results, not just in terms of weight loss, but in how I was feeling and looking every day. I felt stronger, and I could now set, and perhaps realize, reachable goals for weight and performance.

By early October, my weight had dropped another 2 pounds, to 256. At this point, my workouts with Annette were averaging about a 500-calorie burn per session—three cardio intervals of 100 each, plus about 200 for the circuits. That was the good news. Then Annette explained that I needed to have a 3,500-calorie deficit each week to drop 1 pound, so the 500-calorie burn for one workout is the 500-per-day average I needed to achieve that . . . plus eating less in general and increasing my activity on the road—for example, walking more at airports.

More notes on the progress of my workouts:

- Goal is to increase reps to 20 to 25 for variety; increase some weights.

Elliptical	Level 9 increase, and 50 to 55 rpms	did 100 calories, 6:46 minutes
Leg press	55 pounds each side—tough	
Hammer row	50 pounds each side	
Hip extension	10 pounds	
Pushups on knees	20	He looked so much better doing them! His form is so much better, and he did 20!
Oblique crunches with knee lift	10 each side	
Treadmill	8% incline— improvement, 3.5 mph	100 calories = 7 minutes
Lat pulldown	95 pounds— improvement	form is looking good!
Leg extension	90 pounds	he kept saying to raise it, and it feels OK on the knee

Shoulder press	20-pound dumbbell, 10 reps	then 8 reps with 15-pound
Leg curl	60 pounds	
Standing cable rotation	3 plates	
Cable rows in split squat	6 plates	
Hip extension	10 pounds	
This sequence	2 times	
Reverse crunches	20, 15	
Prone hold	11 seconds, 2 times	
Single leg bridge	10, 10	
Seated rotation	10 pounds	15, 10
Elliptical	Level 9, 55 to 57 rpm	107 calories = 7 minutes

RAMPING IT UP: THE QUICKIE

And I then made the decision, with Annette, to try something new. In addition to the regular workouts with Annette, I would add something to the mix. Something called . . . the Quickie. My friend Stephen Pipes, the general manager of the Parker Meridien hotel in New York, had told me about this new program, which he had just installed at Gravity, the health club at the hotel, and he swore by it.

Of course, being a type A personality, I loved the term "Quickie." I had to try it. But one note of caution: "Quickie," as applied by the folks at Gravity, does not equate to "easy."

The motto at Gravity is "It's your workout, not your life." Nevertheless, the Quickie soon became a big part of my life.

I was introduced to Mark Natale, who is the executive director of Gravity and who runs the program. "Your goal may be to lose weight, and that's fine," he explained. "But you can't just depend on tons and tons of cardiovascular work as the answer. While it's absolutely important to overall health, cardiovascular work is not the 'be-all and end-all' to lose weight. In order to really change the shape of your body, you have to incorporate strength training."

Here's where the real confusion starts. I knew that the recommendation for cardiovascular exercise is thirty to sixty minutes, three to five times per week. But the intensity and time for strength exercises are not the same. What Mark taught me—and believe me, I had no clue prior to this—is the difference between cardiovascular aerobic training and anaerobic strength training, and why both are essential—and why they are exact opposites of one another. Strength training sessions should be brief and hard, not long and easy.

Until I met Mark, I had been doing mostly cardiovascular work and functional exercises with Annette. I had lost nearly 30 pounds, but I wanted to lose more. And now, Annette, Mark, and I developed a program that combined my cardiovascular workout with strength training by alternating the two. Whenever I was in New York—about once every four days, for about four days—I spent one session with Annette and one day with Mark.

The Quickie is based on the idea that there is a precise amount of exercise needed to bring about a positive change in your fitness level. It's best to start with the least amount of exercise possible and then see how the body responds.

Essentially, everybody needs the same thing to make his or her body change—and that means you have to push beyond your body's current capabilities. Once you do that, however, you need to rest and allow your body to change. Too many people rush back to the gym and interrupt the process. Or they don't work hard enough to bring about a change.

The Quickie program had me performing nine exercises two times per week. Only one exercise is performed at a time to make one set. I performed that set until I could no longer lift or lower the weight in good form. This is known as *training to failure*. Only one set of each exercise is performed. Why? As Mark explained, "If you perform the set until failure, why do you need another set?" A scary thought, but certainly logical.

"Haven't you exposed the muscle to enough stress to make it change?" Mark continued. "Think of the growth stimulator like a light switch. You don't turn a switch on and off and on and off to get the light on. You switch it on and it's done. The same thing occurs with your muscles. Once they have encountered enough demand, the switch has been thrown. You're done. Move on to the next set."

Another thing that makes the Quickie a completely different approach is the interactive computer screen attached to each machine. Mark set my reps at four-second intervals—and those seconds, as well as the reps, were timed (and recorded) precisely on the computer screen in front of each machine. The goal was to perform each rep so that you didn't complete it in less than four seconds (a total of eight to complete a full rep)—and you couldn't let the weights touch.

With me, Mark focused on two things. First, the speed of each rep. Lift and drop times for the Quickie are four seconds up and four seconds down. Initially, I moved really fast and in a herky-jerky fashion. This is bad for two reasons:

1. That fast motion translates into a lot of momentum, which means it is easy to get hurt. Muscle pulls and strains are common in people who train this way. And to make matters worse . . .
2. I was not really *lifting* the weight. I was essentially throwing it and catching it at different points of the motion. In other words, I was wasting my time, and my muscles were not working as hard as they could have been.

Even if you don't have access to the Quickie computer screen, you can still do the program. Use the same machines, but do the four-secound countdowns on you own.

The second area Mark looked at was my breathing and facial expressions during the workout. Too often, I was holding my breath and contorting my face when the work got really hard. Not good. Both of these things will increase your blood pressure. Mark stood right in front of me, coaching me to breathe at a more normal pace and to relax my face. Easier said than done, but slowly, surely, I began to get into a rhythm.

This was indeed time under tension, and working to failure was—as planned—an inevitability. But it felt good . . .

Annette was there to watch the Quickie, because it also allowed her to note my progress and then adjust the cardio exercises the next day. One important note about the Quickie: It is always done with an instructor, and for an important reason. It is practically impossible for you to push yourself to failure when you are exercising on your own. There's another reason as well. Few gyms are equipped with the Fitlinxx computer link, and it's difficult to duplicate the Quickie on the road. So while the Quickie became an important addition to my exercise routine, my focus had to remain on the cardio with Annette, especially when I would be traveling. But the Quickie was a much needed, and successful, variation in my regime.

So how did I do on the Quickie? I asked Mark to keep a workout journal from the very start.

October 18, 2005

First Workout
Here we go. Let's see how well this guy knows his stuff.

Post-Workout
Went through the nine exercises and got him set up on Fitlinxx. He seems as though he will be fairly strong. Have to focus on the lift and drop time of the weights. This is the area that all people new to the program have to focus on.

Workout Exercise	Weight	Repetitions
Leg press	245	12
Leg curl	40	12
Lat pulldown	125	15
Chest press	80	13
Shoulder press	40	7
Biceps curl	40	11
Triceps extension	30	13
Abdominal crunch	80	14
Lower back extension	85	14

The whole session lasted twenty-four minutes. But then, it was *supposed* to last twenty-four minutes (hence, "the Quickie").

The next day, I could hardly move . . . I needed to rest. And as Mark explained to me, that was not surprising. "Rest is a very important concept that most exercise programs never explain or consider," he said. "After a workout, the body needs to recover the resources that were lost during the workout. Once the body has recovered to its pre-workout state, it can then start the process of growing stronger and fitter, better able to meet the demands of the workout. Most people rush back to the gym before they are ready to and therefore interrupt the change/growth phase. It is really a matter of economics. Think of it like a retirement account. If you are constantly drawing on those savings, you will never realize the effects of compounding interest. Same thing in the gym."

That explains why there is at least one day off between workouts with the Quickie program. And as I became stronger and fitter, I actually needed to *increase* the rest periods! "Becoming stronger means that the inroads into your recovery system are greater and therefore more time needs to elapse between workouts in order to recover and become stronger," Mark explained.

October 20, 2005

Pre-Workout

Now that Peter has been set up on all of the equipment, we can really start to focus on doing the workout perfectly. Have to focus on the speed of the movement and Peter's facial expressions. He has a tendency to hold his breath and grimace, both of which are really bad for blood pressure. He has to be a stoic!

Post-Workout

Great workout! I can see that he will make progress really fast if he sticks with the program.

Workout

Exercise	Weight	Repetitions
Leg press	280	15
Leg curl	60	12
Lat pulldown	155	10
Chest press	100	7
Shoulder press	40	9
Biceps curl	50	13
Triceps extension	50	5*
Abdominal crunch	100	17
Lower back extension	120	15

*Stopped short because of pain in elbow caused by the pad. Need to look at a solution for this.

October 24, 2005

Pre-Workout:

Peter's weights are getting into the range that we want them to be. We are looking for that rep scheme of eight to twelve reps per set. That means he should get at least eight reps and fail before he hits twelve reps. If he does get more than twelve, then I need to increase that weight for the next workout.

Post-Workout

Excellent workout! Peter is really strong, stronger than I realized.

Leg press was at 310 today and still too light.

Leg curl was giving him some knee pain. I have to pay attention to that and work around his knee surgery.

Pulldown was a bit too heavy today. I needed to lighten it up and really work on perfecting that form.

Chest press. Great form. Great tempo. Stay put for the next workout.

Shoulder press. Excellent set. Up two repetitions from last workout with the same weight!

Biceps curl. Very strong and excellent control. Stay put here.

Triceps extension.

Abdominal crunch. Great strength but I need to focus him here to get better control of the weight. He is throwing the weight here rather than lifting it.

Lower back extension. Keep those hips back and in good form.

Workout

Exercise	Weight	Repetitions
Leg press	310	14
Leg curl	65	6*
Lat pulldown	140	13
Chest press	90	9
Shoulder press	40	11
Biceps curl	60	10
Triceps extension	50	2†
Abdominal crunch	125	13
Lower back extension	125	15

*Pain in the knee is limiting his work on this exercise. Monitor and lighten the weight a bit.

†That pad is hurting his elbow and stopping him from doing this. Alternative?

October 26, 2005

Pre-Workout

Late! We were supposed to start at 10:15 A.M. Peter did not arrive until 10:25 A.M. Will have to make him pay a bit.

Post-Workout
Everything went well today. Reduced the weight on the leg curl exercises as a preventative measure for his knee. Weights are up and he is getting it down. Watch some of his form, as he can get sloppy quick!

Workout

Exercise	Weight	Repetitions
Leg press	340	12
Leg curl	40	12
Lat pulldown	155	11
Chest press	90	11
Shoulder press	40	10
Biceps curl	60	11
Triceps extension	50	10
Abdominal crunch	125	13
Lower back extension	140	16

November 7, 2005

Pre-Workout
Late again. . . . The Quickie is perfect for him. How could he have time for anything else? Peter has been traveling for the past ten days and I do not know what he has been doing while he has been away. I am going to scale back his weights to ease him back in. I do not think he has been able to keep up his workouts while traveling. It will be interesting to see how he does today.

Post-Workout
Good workout. Had to ease up a bit today. Probably too little rest on these "business" trips!

Workout

Exercise	Weight	Repetitions
Leg press	320	10
Leg curl	40	12
Lat pulldown	155	13

Chest press	90	11
Shoulder press	40	7
Biceps curl	55	10
Triceps extension	40	10
Abdominal crunch	100	15
Lower back extension	140	10

November 9, 2005

Pre-Workout

Continue pushing Peter after his layoff. I need to make sure he is focusing on the details. Four-second lift, four-second drop, breathing properly, etc. He can get distracted quickly.

Post-Workout

Good progress. Getting back to where he was before the layoff. Had to adjust some range of motion and lift and drop speed issues on the lat pulldown and chest press. His form is perfect now and that is the most important thing. He is about to go away again, so I need to make sure that he can stay consistent.

Workout

Exercise	Weight	Repetitions
Leg press	320	11
Leg curl	50	12
Lat pulldown	155	11
Chest press	90	7
Shoulder press	40	11
Biceps curl	60	8
Triceps extension	50	6
Abdominal crunch	120	12
Lower back extension	125	13

In just six workouts, for a total of approximately 168 minutes (less than three hours of work), Peter lifted almost 74,000 pounds. That's about 440 pounds per minute!

The day following a Quickie, I did my regular routine with Annette. She said I was able to work harder, which is great, and that
when I'm tired I don't talk as much, which is what I want. I
worked hard and was definitely beat. Her notes:

Elliptical	Level 9	8 minutes
Intervals vary between levels 8 and 11; 1 minute hard and 1 minute easy (1:1 ratio)	12 minutes	311 calories total for 20 minutes
Treadmill	3.5 mph; 5.5% incline, 10 minutes	120 calories
Elliptical	steady at Level 11	8 minutes

Annette then took my measurements, and my mood improved dramatically. Since our first meeting, I had lost 2½ inches
around my chest, 6 inches around my waist, and 1¼ inches
around my hips. Not a bad start.

But now it was time to take the exercise program on the
road—and to learn an important travel lesson: that the most important meeting of any trip was the one I make . . . with myself . . . to exercise.

CHAPTER 7

Exercise on the Road

This is, without a doubt, the killer part of the traveler's diet, because it all hinges on your own dependability and determination while you are simultaneously being confronted with a killer travel schedule. This is where people most often fail.

Consider this: In the last decade, the number of U.S. hotels with fitness facilities has grown from 36 percent to 56 percent. And the facilities themselves have dramatically improved. Not too long ago, the words "hotel gym" were an oxymoron. Now, many hotel gyms rival, if not exceed, private fitness centers.

But simply having a great hotel gym doesn't mean you'll use it. The statistics are a little frightening. In almost every piece of research I've seen, travelers rate fitness centers as the most or second most important amenity when traveling. In fact, an overwhelming number of travelers responded that they booked a hotel in large part based on whether it had a fitness center and/or a pool. But the actual utilization rate—how many of the guests actually use the facilities—is a disheartening 6 percent . . . or less.

Still other research indicated reasons why travelers don't use in-house fitness centers. In a survey of three hundred business travelers for Westin Hotels and Resorts, 64 percent said that hotel fitness rooms "seem like an afterthought." And 55 percent said they avoided hotel gyms altogether because they are in bad condition.

And yet enough guests say they want them that the hotels continue to build them. It's bizarre when you think about it, but not to do so—even though so few people use them—would put these hotels at a competitive disadvantage.

Of course, with my schedule, it wasn't a choice, it was a necessity to use hotel fitness centers on the traveler's diet, since so much of my time is spent traveling. Still, bad habits die hard.

My first question—and a dangerous one—was how little exercise could I get away with on the road? And that, of course had to be considered in the context of all the other moments of abuse travelers experience—along with strange cities, strange hotels, strange beds, and strange sleep patterns.

Luckily, my fitness regime on the road *was* maintained because, before I would fly anywhere, I'd find out whether the hotel had a fitness center and/or a trainer. If the hotel had a fitness center *and* a trainer, it was easy. I'd simply send an e-mail about my cardio and weight protocols to the hotel and arrange to be taken immediately to the hotel gym the moment I checked in—no detours or diversions.

It's a matter of how well you know yourself. Remember, part of making the traveler's diet work is understanding that we don't change our lifestyle when we change our location. In my case, I recognized that, given the chance, I would easily revert to those bad patterns. Left on my own, I'd just check in to my hotel room and go immediately to my BlackBerry or log on to the Internet. But my new approach is to get the exercise out of the way first. And if the hotel doesn't have a trainer, the concierge can get me one. And if there are no trainers, I also have a protocol for exercising by myself in my room. But either way, the hotel would be ready for me—or I would be ready for myself.

Over a year-long period, I carried out this plan in more than forty cities—in a host of chain hotels such as Sheratons, Marriotts, and Hiltons, as well as in individual hotels like the Broadmoor in Colorado Springs and the Atlantic in Fort Lauderdale, and even on the Celebrity cruise ship *Summit*.

Each hotel gym was different, of course, but I was able to adapt much, if not all, of Annette Lang's training regime at every location. Frequently, both the trainer and I had to improvise when the equipment wasn't quite the same. But the important thing is that the plan *worked*!

My first attempt at trying to exercise on the road took place on a quick two-day trip to Kansas City, where I had a reservation at the Marriott. But I needed a workout there as well. The hotel had not only a health club, but also a trainer. I was in luck.

Annette e-mailed the hotel with exactly what was needed to keep me on track:

- A full-body routine, for one hour, was the goal. The objective was to get as much movement in as possible.

- No squats or lunges yet—to protect the right knee from further damage to an old ACL injury.

- The focus was to be on free weights, cable, and machines—using whatever was available in the facility.

- Three cardio intervals at moderate-high intensity for five minutes each were to be included.

- The workout format was to be a circuit, whereby I would do one round of exercises with a cardiovascular interval, then change the exercises the next round, if possible.

- The trainer was to encourage me to be more active in general during this visit to the city.

Workout

The goal was fifteen reps for each exercise—not "to failure," though. I would start with cardio for five to ten minutes. Then I would do another cardio interval for five to eight minutes in between circuits. My goal was to get through two to three circuits. Annette provided suggestions for substitutions in case the hotel's health club didn't have the equipment. The circuits consisted of the following exercises.

Circuit 1
- Elliptical Life Fitness, Manual Level 8, at least 50 rpm, five minutes.

- Straight-arm cable pulldown, 70 pounds. Substitute some kind of pulling exercise; try to get different angles.

- Biceps curls into overhead presses with 15-pound dumbbells.

- Cable core rotations, standing, with three plates. Hold the grips with both hands, arms straight at midsection height, and rotate, letting the legs move with the rotation. (Substitute rotation with dumbbell or medicine ball.)

- Leg press if available, 45 pounds each side.

- Dead lifts, with 15-pound dumbbells. I needed to work on my form, learning to move from the hips and not the spine.

- If the hotel gym had a slant board, I could lean on it to do hip extensions, with a 10-pound dumbbell held out in front.

Circuit 2
- Treadmill, manual mode, five minutes, at least 7 percent incline, 3 miles per hour.

- Lat pulldown, 80 pounds. (Substitute a pulling exercise.)

- Leg curl, 40 pounds. (Substitute dead lifts or bridges.)

- Leg extension, 60 pounds.

- Reverse fly, machine, 40 pounds. (Substitute cable; pull with elbows out to side.)

- Single-arm cable row with opposite leg in front, three plates. (Substitute rows with dumbbells or machine.)

- Twelve pushups on knees; keep head in line with body.

- Reverse crunches.

- Stability ball bridges—hold ball to keep stable. (Substitute bridges on floor.)

- Lateral holds on knees, eight seconds. Lie on side on forearm; keep elbow right under shoulder, body in straight line, with knees bent. Lift up hips and hold.

- Reverse crunches.

Circuit 3
- Elliptical; same as before.

- Do one of the preceding circuits or something different, depending on the equipment available.

As soon as I checked in, shortly after 3 P.M., I was introduced to trainer Monique McDaniel. And she took me directly to the gym, wasting no time in putting me through Annette's paces, not to mention a few of her own. As I had done in New York with Annette, I asked Monique to keep a diary of my progress:

Peter was open to my suggestion of modifying a few of the exercises by integrating a stability ball and a balance dome (I brought my own). My training is centered around the core and instability because I believe in the benefits one gets from ball work not only as a trainer but also from my clients. It is the one piece of equipment that when you use it you feel immediate work on your muscles. My philosophy in training is to strengthen from the inside out, and one effective way to do this is to use as much in stability props as possible. I explained my training background and philosophy and told him to be prepared to feel the "quivva" sensation, that tingling feeling deep in the abdominal muscles when the muscles are contracted from doing abdominal work on the ball and on the balance dome. I saw his eagerness, and with thumbs up, we began.

Immediately, I was aware that Peter has been working with a professional trainer because of his breathing techniques and his initial approach to each exercise. He knew how to hold the free weights properly and waited patiently to hear my direction for the momentum needed when pushing and or pulling the weight. We started with a general warm-up on the elliptical machine at a medium resistance. He was quick to tell me he did not stay on there long; an average of six to eight minutes was all he wanted to do. I wasn't surprised by this because I find many people dislike cardio work regardless of whether it is a warm-up or a full twenty- to thirty-minute workout. Once off the elliptical, I had him sit on a 65-centimeter stability ball and took him through general stretches to loosen up his total body. Next I did a balance assessment by having him lift one knee at a time while raising the opposite arm. This is a general assessment to see how balanced a person is while sitting on an unstable surface. I was impressed that he did not waver much on the ball and did not fall off; his balance was good.

After the stretching, I had him do balance and stability work while standing on the balance dome. This, he found, was a bit tricky and I had to assist by standing in front of him with arms out just in case he tilted too much forward and fell off. Peter did well once I encouraged him to focus on his midsection for balance. He did a couple of side-to-side shifts on the ball, warming up his hips and thighs.

Once off the dome, we followed Annette's routine with just a couple of modifications. His program included lat pulldowns to work his upper back muscles. We did a set with the machine and one set while on the ball. While he was seated on the ball, I guided Peter to tilt back, relaxing into the ball and engaging his lower abdominals while pulling the bar to his sternum. This can be a challenging move if one is alone in the gym, because you have to grab the bar from above and position the ball accordingly to walk out and tilt. Peter liked this modification because he was working multiple muscles with one move. He said he could feel his lower abdominals working with each pull of the bar, and this was a good sign. For his lower body, Annette had him do leg extensions using the leg extension machine with 30 to 40 pounds. I made a slight modification by having Peter do leg extensions using his own body weight and balance by sitting on the ball, extending one leg out at a time and holding for four counts. I also included leg curls with the ball. This move, I believe, works the hamstrings a bit deeper and you don't have to do as many repetitions. We ended the session with yoga stretches on the ball, an assisted stretch, and standard crunches.

The next session forced us to improvise, but also taught me some on-the-road options. It was scheduled for 6:15 the next morning. But when I got to the hotel gym, it was a Saturday, and it was closed.

So we headed to the elevator and out the lobby doors, for a long predawn walk through downtown Kansas City.

Monique's notes:

> We went down 10th Street, then turned and traveled west to the Quality Hill District, a nice area with several brownstone apartments and condominiums. We had a couple of inclines to attack, which Peter did fine, and his conversation never wavered. I was the active listener to the refreshing conversation and also kept a keen eye on his gait, pelvic tilt, and core engagement.
>
> I watched Peter's cadence and listened for any abnormal breathing to make sure the pace was a good one. A couple of times I reminded Peter to relax his shoulders and soften his knees while walking uphill. Once back at the hotel, we found a set of stairs between the lobby and the mezzanine, and I had him do two to four heel raises per step. There were about twenty-five steps. This increased his heart rate a bit and worked his calves. He did this twice, and at the top we found a bench to do general stretches. With both feet extended, legs straight, I had him reach slowly forward while rounding his back to touch his toes. He didn't get to his toes, however. I told him that, with daily stretching, in about a month's time he should be able to touch the top of his shoes. After stretching, I had him do balance/stability work with the balance dome that I have with me at all times. A benefit of having the dome is its compact size. This small air-inflated cushion is the best thing around, designed to improve lower back health by offering a constant stimulation while sitting on it or using it to assist with several core exercises. We didn't need much space, and he was

comfortable on the mezzanine-level floor. While he sat with knees bent, I had him slowly roll back onto the balance dome and hold for eight counts. This was an excellent low back and abdominal exercise, and after a few of those he was feeling, and I was seeing, the quivva! He did several standard back exercises such as this one: While on hands and knees with dome under one knee, he extended one arm at a time, holding for a few counts, and then alternated with opposite knee and arm. Peter also did many challenging lower body moves such as alternate leg lifts with the dome under his tailbone and pelvic bridges. This session ended with standing work on the dome, assisted stretches, and modified yoga moves.

Session 3—Sunday, 7:15 A.M.

For a change of scenario, Peter met me at my midtown training studio promptly at 7:15 A.M. I had Peter start with the elliptical for a warm-up and then explained he would do interval training for the first thirty minutes and then end with core training. He did a leg circuit using the leg extension, leg curl, and seated calf machines. Between each set he was on the elliptical for three minutes, medium to high resistance, and did a set of twenty-five crunches on the ball. Once that was completed, I brought out all the instability devices of choice. I had Peter stand on the BOSU ball, a dome device on one side and a flat surface on the other. While balancing on the dome, he did biceps curls, side lateral shoulder lifts, triceps rope pulldowns, and shoulder shrugs. All of these upper body moves also worked his core and several stabilizer muscles. Then he was on the foam roller, a tube device made out of hard Styrofoam. I had him straddle the roller and sit down. Once he was comfortable sitting up, I had him roll back slowly until his head, neck, and shoulders were flat on the roller and his spine was aligned. I instructed him to engage his abdominal muscles and slowly lift his leg up and bend his knee to his chest, holding for eight counts, then relax and do the other leg. This is a great lower abdominal exercise. Next, with both knees to his chest, he dropped his heels for four counts and then came back to start. It didn't take too many of these before he felt and I saw the quivva. He did a set of alternate leg lifts, both bent-knee and straight, and minicrunches. Next, I placed a small, cushioned 3-pound ball at his tailbone and had him roll back and hold that position for eight counts. Again, it did not take too many of those before he felt the shaking of his midsection and a grimace was on his face. The session was complete with an assisted stretch on the massage table and a minimassage from a therapeutic stick. This is a bendable stick with ridges used to relax muscles.

Thanks in no small part to Monique, I now look for stairs whenever possible. And yes, when I do those crunches, I feel the "quivva."

Over the next nine months, wherever I traveled—from Orlando to Amman, Jordan; from Chicago to Bangkok—I sought out the trainers at hotel gyms. And I never had a bad experience.

In Fort Lauderdale, at the Atlantic Hotel, I worked with trainer Norman Sarmiento, and in one nonstop hour, he had me do thirty minutes on the elliptical, then leg squats with free weights and squats using the Swiss ball, followed by Annette's program, using biceps machines, upper chest presses, and the full routine. Norman followed this with abdominal exercises using the Swiss ball (fifty reps). On my second day, he repeated everything from the first day, and then bumped up the elliptical machine to Level 14 for two-minute intervals, followed after fifteen minutes by two series of twenty reps of leg squats with free weights, shoulders with free weights, and biceps on the bench, for two series of twelve reps. And just when I thought we were done, he had me do fifty abdominal reps on the Swiss ball and to finish, fifteen minutes on the treadmill at 10° slant and 3.5 miles per hour.

In California, I met trainer David Dorian-Ross at the Montage Resort and Spa in Laguna Beach. It's tough to find a better view from a hotel fitness center, but the workouts are intense. David watched carefully as I did my elliptical workout for thirty minutes—he was checking for posture (abs in, chin up, and shoulder blades down), as well as making sure that my feet were parallel. He made me use my muscles and not just rely on the foot pedals to keep me in position.

Also, he kept me working in the medium-intensity range, well below the anaerobic threshold—the point at which you are no longer working with oxygen, which is often signaled by not being able to walk and talk without gasping a little for air! He also monitored my heart rate, and was impressed (me, too) that it stayed at a consistent 130 beats per minute. One of the things I've now been able to master is getting on my treadmill at my Los Angeles home at 6 A.M., ramping it up to 3.7 miles per hour at a ten degree incline, and making my early morning calls to the East Coast, without anyone suspecting (until they read this book) that I was on the treadmill!

David then worked with me on assisted stretch exercises. He's a firm believer in making flexibility training a part of your regular routine, especially for frequent travelers. Not only will it mitigate any of the normal aches and pains of travel, but being more flexible also significantly reduces the risk of injury and makes you stronger. In particular, he worked on my lower back muscles, hamstrings, calves, piriformis, and glutes. Why?

He chose these muscles specifically because when these are stretched, it is easier to do the abdominal core work that comes next.

We did two specific ab exercises, and here's a little surprise: When we were finished, David told me we had been doing basic Pilates! Turns out he's a Pilates master and believes it's the most concise and effective form of abdominal training.

As he explained it to me, the basic posture of Pilates starts with the breath. Breathe in through the nose and out through the mouth. On exhale, make it throaty and loud, as if you are trying to fog a mirror. First, pull in your lower abs (what all men do when they're at the beach and a cute girl walks by—really: It's a genetic impulse). Inhale, and as you exhale, flatten down your rib cage (biomechanically, you are contracting your oblique muscles, which attach at the rib cage and the hips).

The first Pilates exercise we did was a hip lift, which is properly called "the pelvic peel." Inhale, exhale, flatten ribs, and—using your ab strength only!—lift your hips into the air, peeling your spine off the floor one vertebra at a time. At the highest lift point, inhale again, then exhale (flatten your ribs again), and slowly peel the spine back down on the floor again. Keep pulling those abs in as you go down!

The second Pilates exercise we did was a crunch (called by Pilates people, "the chest lift"). This time your hips stay down on the floor, and the head and shoulders come off the ground. Inhale, exhale, flatten rib cage, and pull the abs in. Let the power of your abdominal contraction pull you up into the crunch. Here is the add-on we did: At the top of the crunch, inhale and reach your hands to the outside of one thigh. As you exhale, let the lower hand pull you higher while the upper hand pulls you into a bit of a twist. Remember, you don't have to come up too high—just keep focusing on the integrity of the ab contraction! Inhale again, and bring your hands behind your head again. Then exhale and lower down slowly.

Pilates was certainly a different experience for me, but it did teach me to breathe in a new way.

Speaking of breathing, I had to adjust to a different kind of workout—at a different altitude—in Colorado Springs, at the Broadmoor. I wanted to do the same routines on the machines, but fitness supervisor Brian Newman wanted me to drink more water—and a lot of it—before and during the exercise circuit, because of the altitude. And he was right. My heart rate zoomed to 147 on the elliptical—well within range, but the difference was definitely noticeable. And I needed that water.

Over the course of a year, I repeated this gym/trainer routine in many hotels on my trips. And it always made the difference.

But what about the hotels with no trainers?

Annette Lang devised a plan for that as well. But it required me to be disciplined enough to use the gyms and follow her program. I must admit that I didn't do as well here. While I used the gym, I didn't follow her routines as well—or as much—as I should have. Instead, I found myself doing thirty minutes on the ellipticals and fifteen on the treadmills. But *something* was definitely better than what I had been doing before—nothing.

And then came the killer: the hotels with no trainers *and* no fitness center.

Here's where improvisation saves the day. This is what you can do in your hotel room, using just the furniture in the room and the luggage you brought with you.

As many of you know, I believe there are two kinds of airline bags: carry-on . . . and lost. So the exercise program I use in my hotel room involves those carry-on bags, usually full of mail and magazines (and averaging about 20 to 25 pounds each). It also includes dresser drawers, chairs, and closet doors, as well as the telephone directory and, of course, the bed.

Let's start with a dresser drawer. Remove it and place it upside down on the floor, and then use it for one-leg squats, as well as for lunges.

Next, a chair. I put the chair against a wall facing out, then use it for triceps dips: I hold the end of the chair, with my fingers facing forward, then slide my butt off the chair and lower myself down, for about ten reps.

The phone book comes in handy as a free weight to raise above my head. And if I'm feeling particularly motivated, I use the desk. I've already moved the chair away, so I slide under the desk and use it for table chin-ups. I use the closet door for wall sits.

Then I turn to the bed. It's my exercise bench. Using my carry-on bags, and alternating sides, I do one-arm rows with the suitcases. I can also do lifts with the bags (upright rows). I can do many of the lifts, curls, and presses that I might normally do with free weights and get the same effect, simply by using the edge of my bed as my bench and putting one knee on the edge of the bed and one leg on the floor, then repeating many of Annette's exercises.

And I can do all of this while watching Leno! Who knew?

Using the desk chair in my hotel room (if it's not on wheels), I can do many of my stretching exercises:

- *A simple squat.*   You can hold something up over your head to make it more challenging, such as a phone book, your backpack, or even a chair.

- *Jump squats.*   Just jump in the air a little bit and land quietly in a squat. Then jump up again. If you do the jump squat first, you need less weight for the other exercises, as you will be tired.

- *Walking lunges.*   Start at the door. Take a step forward, bend both knees so that you get ninety-degree angles at the knees, stand back up, and take a step forward with the other leg. You can hold something in each hand or hold something in front of you—a water bottle, for example.

- *Squats with rotations.*   Place your backpack or duffel bag or other object on the outside of your left foot. Squat down, pick up the object, and lift it along a diagonal line, up toward your right shoulder, as if you were going to put it on a shelf. Then switch sides.

- *Pushups.*   Do them with your hands on the desk, on a chair, or on the floor, depending on your preferred level of difficulty (closer to the floor is harder). You can do them on your knees on the floor, too.

- *Rows.*   Use a duffel bag or backpack. Stand with one hand on the back of a chair; lean over from the hip, keeping the natural curve in your lower back. Hold the bag in one hand with arm straight down toward the floor. Pull your elbow up to the ceiling as you lift the bag. Pull shoulders down and back relative to you as you pull.

- *Core rotations.*   Sit on the floor with your legs in front of you and your knees bent. Lean back slightly, holding something light in both hands, and rotate your upper body from side to side.

- *Supermans.*   Lie facedown with your arms by your ears. Lift up both arms and both legs at the same time.

In general, when you travel, here are some things to consider:

- Use the stairs whenever possible; it really does make a difference! Especially after a flight, it will make you feel much better and less groggy.

- If you do even a short workout at the beginning of the day, you will feel better and get yourself in the right mind-set, which might help you to avoid overeating throughout the rest of the day.

- Plan a walking tour of the city you are in to incorporate more movement into your sightseeing.

- Prepare by bringing along things like good shoes and enough clothing to avoid sabotaging your own efforts! (I know this problem all too well—in the past, I avoided working out because I hadn't packed shorts or sneakers. Obviously, this no longer happens. These are now the very first things I pack.)

If all else fails, just be creative. And be honest with yourself. If you're not a morning person, you're not going to walk in the morning. Take a walk after dinner instead. And it doesn't have to be a traditional power walk, either. For example, here's a small but interesting statistic: a University of Missouri-Columbia study looked at dog owners who started walking their puppies for ten minutes each day. After a year, the dog owners recorded an average 14-pound weight loss! What does that have to do with travel and hotels? At some hotels, like the Ritz-Carlton in Bachelor Gulch, Colorado, they will actually loan you a golden retriever for the day or evening. And that spells . . . an opportunity to get out and walk the dog, or in the case of the dog I got when I was at the hotel, the dog walks *you*.

And then I discovered the BodyRev. Now available at a growing number of Marriotts (call downstairs and they'll deliver one to your room), it's an amazing portable exercise device—a small machine with spinning interior wheels and handles.

The BodyRev was developed by Alden Mills, a former U.S. Navy SEAL who believes that, in his case, necessity was definitely the mother of invention. Mills was a platoon commander in 1995. "Back then the SEAL teams found we had to make a fundamental shift in the way we did training," he relates. "We used to use age-old bodybuilding principles—that is, work from the outside in. We worked on certain muscle groups, in the arms . . . your biceps, triceps . . . or in the legs . . . and eventually we'll get to the abdominals. What ended up happening over time is that the injury rate started climbing in SEAL teams and we had to figure out a better way to train. We had these big hulking macho guys that had very weak core strength. And . . . we really flipped our paradigm to functional training. Suddenly, more muscles engage at the same time, which means more calories burn, which means more blood flow, which means heart rate goes up. So now I get to tone, tighten, and burn fat . . . *while* I get to do movement patterns that better simulate things I do in life, which could then result in less injury."

The challenge was that in the exercise and fitness world, there weren't any pieces of equipment that simulated objects you would pick up in real life. If you think about it, you will realize that the weight of almost anything you lift in life is in the center of the object, and the handles are on the outside, so that you hold it in front of you. Very few objects are carried using a bar across your shoulders.

Thus, the genesis of the BodyRev concept came from the idea of high-repetition, low-weight movement patterns, which can be adjusted to any age or fitness level, while combining cardio and strength training at the same time.

The BodyRev proved to me that fitness doesn't have to be difficult, and it doesn't have to use big and bulky equipment. This is a simple machine, with two free-spinning handles that adapt to the way you move. That sounds easy enough—until you pick it up and use it.

The BodyRev workout lasts just fifteen minutes, but your heart rate goes up right away. In less than four minutes, you're sweating, and before you know it, four sets of abdominals, your lower back muscles, and your spinal muscles are simultaneously engaged in the exercise. If you extend your hands in front of your torso, your core is also naturally engaged. Once you lower down to a squat, you're going to engage all the major muscle groups at the same time. And when that happens, I guarantee you that you are going to feel it in your legs, your buttocks, and your arms—and in your core. Then there's the calorie burn— about 250 calories in a fifteen-minute regimen.

"The biggest problem with exercise on the road," Mills says, "is that people want to get cardio so they can burn fat and they want to get muscle conditioning . . . strengthening, so they can also tone. Combine the two of those together and you'll get a terrific endorphin rush that will get you going throughout the rest of the day. But to put both of those together at the same time requires a lot of time and up until now, a lot of different pieces of equipment." Until the BodyRev came along, that is.

You can find the equipment in many hotel gyms and fitness centers, but finding the time to use it and the person to walk you through the workout can be another challenge. I planned ahead whenever possible and asked on-site trainers to help me.

The beauty of the BodyRev is that it's all low impact. And it's all available . . . in your hotel room.

MORE GYM/FITNESS SERVICES AT HOTELS

Here are some additional ways to maintain your workout regimen when you are traveling.

Marriott's Fit For You

You can find the BodyRev at the Marriott, where you can also borrow equipment such as the Body Wedge 21 and the Traveling Trainer. The Fit for You culinary program complements the fitness focus with room service and catering items that are carb-conscious, low-fat, and low-cholesterol.

Following the success of its Renaissance ClubSport in Walnut Creek, California, and to cater to guests who take exercising very seriously, Marriott plans to open fifteen new ClubSport locations nationwide over the next five to seven years. With 23,000 square feet of cardio, circuit, and weight equipment, the Renaissance ClubSport in Walnut Creek also has a basketball gym, racquetball and squash courts, and swimming pools, and offers yoga, step, cycling, Pilates, and tai chi classes. ClubSport has over nine thousand local members, but hotel guests are given complimentary access to all ClubSport facilities and classes. (http://marriott.com)

Hilton/Bally Total Fitness

Hilton and Bally have teamed up to offer several different travel fitness options for your stay. A Bally personal trainer will either come to the hotel or meet you at a local Bally location. You can rent an in-room treadmill for a nominal fee or purchase the Travel Fit Kit, which comes with a pair of 5-pound dumbbells, a resistant tube for upper body conditioning, elastic bands for leg exercises, a yoga mat, and a simple exercise booklet to guide you through your in-room workout.

Westin WORKOUT, Powered by Reebok

Every Westin WORKOUT Room allows guests to maintain their fitness regime by working out in the privacy of their own room. In-room features include a Reebok Tomahawk XL Indoor Cycle or Life Fitness Treadmill, Reebok Pilates/Yoga and Spinning DVDs, and a custom-designed fitness shelf that holds adjustable dumbbells, resistance tubing, a stability ball, a yoga mat, and additional Reebok workout equipment. This convenient, private exercise environment also features a Rodale fitness library that includes *Runner's World* magazine, a local running map, *Bicycling Magazine,* and complimentary bottled water.

The Westin Chicago River North offers a No Excuse Workout plan whereby the hotel provides freshly laundered workout clothes (T-shirts, shorts, and even sneakers) for guests who have forgotten to pack their own workout gear. The No Excuse Workout plan is perfect for travelers looking to pack light but who still want to stay fit while they are on vacation. The hotel even has a licensed personal trainer on call to provide complimentary sessions for guests throughout the day. (www .westinchicago.com)

Stay Fit at Hyatt

Hyatt Hotels and Resorts now offers a selection of workout offerings for the fitness-conscious travelers staying at their hotels across North America and the Caribbean. In addition to upgraded cardio and strength equipment, they offer:

- YogaAway—televised in-room yoga sessions. Guests can choose from energizing, calming, or strengthening routines. At select Hyatt hotels and resorts, like Spa Avania in Scottsdale, Arizona, Hyatt offers scheduled yoga classes and private yoga sessions with YogaAway-sanctioned instructors. These sessions are offered at times convenient for business travelers.

- A Stay Fit Concierge is on call at Hyatt properties to offer Apparel-on-Demand, which provides exercise wear, within an hour of receiving a request, for travelers who prefer to pack light.

- GPS Forerunner system to allow runners and walkers to monitor their heart rate and distance (as well as helping them find their way back to the hotel).

(http://goldpassport.hyatt.com)

Kimpton Hotels "Om Away From Home"

Guests can really relax during their stay with the "Om Away From Home" program at Kimpton Hotels. Yoga instruction is made easy and accessible to guests through the Yoga Channel offered on in-room television sets free of charge. A complimentary basket filled with essential yoga equipment by Gaiam (a wellness company that specializes in yoga and meditation products), including a yoga mat, block, and strap, is available to guests during their stay. The basket also includes the most recent issue of *Yoga Journal* magazine, a leading authority on all things yoga. (www.kimptonlifewellness.com)

Estancia La Jolla Hotel and Spa

Estancia is a combination luxury resort and spa with conference center. So even if you're on a business trip, you can go outside to get fit. Outdoor fitness options include Saturday sunrise yoga classes in the outdoor garden; guided hikes through the coastal La Jolla terrain that incorporate a variety of fitness elements including cardio and plyometric training; sea kayaking through San Diego's famous underwater reserve, where you can build up those arm muscles while watching bottlenose dolphins, sea lions, leopard sharks, and bat rays; and the La Jolla bike tour, which gives you a cardio workout as you bike through La Jolla and nearby towns. (www.estancialajolla.com)

FINDING YOUR GYM AWAY FROM HOME

If you travel often and find that hotel gyms just don't cut it, check to see if your home gym allows you to use their branches in the cities where you will be traveling. If you belong to a large gym network, there's usually just a nominal fee to work out at one of their other locations, and sometimes it's free. For frequent travelers, this can be a convenient way to exercise your body—and your gym membership.

If you belong to a private club, see whether it's a member of the International Health, Racquet & Sportsclub Association. If so, you may be able to use another IHRSA club in the area you plan to visit, for free.

Member of the YMCA? If so, you may have reciprocity privileges for free as well. The rules vary from state to state, but in Virginia, for example, any visiting YMCA member can use Virginia YMCA facilities—just by presenting an out-of-state membership card.

Two of the nation's largest chains, 24 Hour Fitness and Bally, offer membership levels that permit you to use their fitness centers anywhere in the country. Membership fees vary depending on where you live, and promotions change regularly. As an example, 24 Hour Fitness in the L.A. area has a plan for just under $40 per month that gives you access to all 24 Hour Fitness locations nationwide.

- International Health, Racquet & Sportsclub Association (http://cms.ihrsa.org)

- YMCA of America (www.ymca.net)

- 24 Hour Fitness (www.24hourfitness.com)

- Bally Total Fitness (www.ballytotalfitness.com)

How to Find a Gym Overseas

Doing a little homework before you arrive at your destination can be invaluable if you are trying to locate a gym in a foreign country. If you're a member of an American gym chain—especially one with international locations—an upgraded membership can include usage at international locations. Your American location should be able to help you find gyms abroad, too—after all, the same exercise chain will probably have different names in different countries. In Asia, for example, 24 Hour Fitness is known as California Gyms or California Fitness.

These are the three gym chains with the most international locations:

- *24 Hour Fitness (as California Gyms):* This is the smallest but fastest-growing chain internationally. As California Gyms, the company is now a significant presence in Hong Kong, Malaysia, Taiwan, Singapore, and Thailand, in addition to several locations in Canada. (www.24hourfitness.com)

- *Gold's Gym:* This is the largest and most prominent chain nationally and internationally, with over 550 locations in over two dozen countries, including more than a dozen in Canada, eighteen in Japan, ten in India, and sixteen in Mexico. (www.goldsgym.com)

- *World Gym:* You can find a few dozen in various countries, mostly in Latin America, Eastern Europe, and the Middle East. (www.worldgym.com)

If you're going to be in a foreign city for an extended period, consider purchasing a short-term membership at a local gym. Many cities have popular and interesting chains that are unique to them, and a little Googling before you arrive should enable you to find one. Chains such as Paris's Gymnase Clubs will let you exercise at a number of locations around the city—a big bonus if your itinerary has you racing all over the city. Alternatively, ask your hotel's concierge for a recommendation of a local chain or club.

Non–chain members should look for International Health, Racquet and Sportsclub Association affiliates, which offer discounts to members of other IHRSA gyms. If you're a member of an American gym that's in the IHRSA, you'll be able to get an IHRSA-valid membership card for an additional fee on top of your regular membership. Abroad, this means you'll have to pay a nominal visitor's fee instead of the usually much higher day-pass fee. (http://cms.ihrsa.org)

CHAPTER 8

The Traveler's Diet . . . at Sea

I don't care what anyone says . . . you will never lose weight on a cruise ship—unless, of course, you contract the Norwalk-like virus and are sick throughout your cruise.

Assuming you won't be confined to your cabin while you have an extended conversation on the porcelain telephone, you will be confronted with food. Everywhere, anywhere, and almost anytime. At last count, I think there were forty-seven separate meals per day served on every single cruise ship. I exaggerate, of course, but not by much.

And if you think people are eating a lot at sea, you're probably underestimating their actual intake.

Consider this: In the first year since the massive, 150,000-ton *Queen Mary 2* was in service, cruise-line officials discovered, much to their surprise, that some of the furniture was breaking. In fact, dozens of chairs on the liner collapsed—under the weight of obese American passengers!

"Our passengers are much heavier than we planned for," one crew member told England's *Daily Mail* newspaper. "And we do have ten restaurants on the ship, so if they are big when they get on, they are bigger when they get off."

Now that's a nightmare marketing motto for any cruise line.

But cruise lines are now enjoying huge passenger growth in another sense as well. More than eight million passengers went on cruises from North American ports in 2003. Over ten million people worldwide travel on cruise ships each year.

For overweight people, cruises are both a blessing and a curse. As more ships leave from more ports in North America—making them a drive-to destination—obese or overweight people are spared the embarrassment of trying to fit into an airline seat to go on their vacation. But the temptations they are faced with at sea are often too much to refuse.

Last year, I took a seven-day cruise aboard the Celebrity cruise ship *Summit*. And the numbers—as they related to food consumed—were nothing short of staggering. In one seven-day circuit, the passengers on board consumed the following:

- 24,236 pounds of beef
- 7,216 pounds of pork
- 1,680 pounds of sausage
- 2,100 pounds of lobster
- 15,150 pounds of potatoes
- 600 quarts of ice cream
- 240 gallons of cream
- 5,750 pounds of sugar
- 450 pounds of jelly
- 1,936 pounds of cookies

And let's not forget the alcohol:

- 3,400 bottles of wine
- 10,100 bottles of beer

Is the ship listing heavily to port yet? It might as well be. The average person gains 8 pounds on a seven-day cruise.

For me, the challenge was not to lose weight on my cruise—it was just to not gain any. Toward that end, I followed this regimen.

SKIP THE BUFFETS

Eat meals at regular intervals, and smaller portions. Buffets on board cruise ships often turn into feeding frenzies. Some cruise lines, like Celebrity, have special spa areas, where spa cuisine is available all day. These dishes are put on the plate for you, so you won't have to do the portion sizing. (Translation: The food is not spilling over the edge of the plate, as it is when I finish at most buffets!)

And definitely skip the midnight buffets. In the past, my eating behavior on board cruise ships was outrageous—if it was there, I had to have it.

These days, I follow the same routine on a cruise ship as on shore: I drink one 16-ounce, or two 8-ounce, bottles of water about 11 P.M., and I have an apple. That's all I need on shore—and that's all I need on the ship.

EATING RIGHT ON BOARD

Here are some tips about how to eat right on the ship and some guidance on the cruise lines that offer you light eating options.

Let's be absolutely honest here. No one in their right mind goes on a cruise to lose weight. If we're lucky—really lucky—we can, if we do it right, go on a cruise and actually *maintain* our current weight. The ADA's Cynthia Sass has a formula that works for weight maintenance on cruises. Allow yourself to consume

- 10 calories per pound of your body weight if you are sedentary or overweight

- 13 calories per pound of your body weight for low activity level (see below), or after the age of fifty-five

- 15 calories per pound of your body weight for moderate activity (see below)

- 18 calories per pound of your body weight for strenuous activity (see below)

Activity Levels:

- *Low activity:* No planned, regular daily physical activity; occasional weekend or recreational activities such as golf

- *Moderate activity:* Thirty to sixty minutes of physical activity like swimming, jogging, or fast walking most days of the week

- *Strenuous activity:* Sixty minutes or more of vigorous physical activity such as spinning class, racquetball, or the like, most days of the week

So a 165-pound adult with a low activity level needs about 2,145 calories to maintain his or her current weight.

If you're trying to lose weight on this trip, you should create a 500-calorie deficit per day by cutting 250 calories from your food intake and burning 250 calories through physical activity. *(Note: Eliminating too many calories can cause you to lose water and muscle weight, slow down your metabolism, and increase your risk of injuries. It can also result in irritability, mood swings, and cravings, causing you to rebound binge-eat.)* Thus, a 165-pound person can aim for a total calorie intake of about 1,900 per day (250 less than what's needed to maintain current weight), or about 630 per meal, and if the person walks briskly for a total of thirty-five minutes each day, it will burn an additional 250 calories.

However, be careful not to overestimate the rate at which you burn calories. As in our example here, a 165-pound adult has to walk briskly for thirty-five minutes to burn just 250 calories. Many people are more active on a cruise than they might be at home, so they feel as if they're burning lots more calories and can afford to indulge—this is a big mistake.

Here are some additional calculations to help you gauge how fast you burn calories. A 200-pound person (male or female) burns roughly

- 300 calories during a fifty-minute tai chi class

- 320 calories during a fifty-minute water aerobics class

- 400 calories during a fifty-minute yoga class

- 450 calories in a fifty-minute aerobics class

- 340 calories doing fifty minutes of ballroom dancing

- 440 calories walking briskly for fifty minutes

- 460 calories doing fifty minutes of disco dancing

- 520 calories when weight training for fifty minutes

- 610 calories playing tennis for fifty minutes (singles)

- 670 calories when swimming for fifty minutes

A 200-pound person would burn 105 calories if he or she walked 1 mile at a 3-mile-per-hour pace. The number of calories burned during a 1-mile walk depends on the person's speed and body weight.

Watch your alcohol intake. Alcohol can cause weight gain in three major ways. First, it's an appetite stimulant. Second, it causes you to lose your inhibitions and allows you to make menu choices you wouldn't make if you were sober. And finally, it's the mixers that'll get you. Sour mix, cream, cola, and the like, can add several hundred calories. If you do drink, follow these guidelines:

- Choose wine, a wine spritzer, light beer, or a mixed drink with a calorie-free mixer such as club soda, water, or diet soda, which have the fewest calories.

- Drink an 8-ounce glass of water between alcoholic drinks. This helps prevent dehydration, thus reducing your chance of having a hangover the next day, but it also helps reduce your total alcohol intake.

- Keep in mind that a 12-ounce light beer (standard bottle), 5 ounces of wine (about the size of a small fruit cup), or a 1.5-ounce shot (shot glass) equals about 100 calories each, and each of these is considered one drink. The 2005 Dietary Guidelines recommend restricting your intake to one drink a day for women, and two for men.

Use the buddy system to keep yourself on track diet-wise when you travel, or take preventative measures. If you're going on the cruise with every intention of adhering to your fitness and nutrition goals, and your significant other has every intention of throwing caution to the wind, pigging out, and being a boat potato, you may be in trouble. There's a way to handle a significant other who doesn't support your healthy eating and exercise goals. If you are going on a cruise, you can plan to go with another couple so you have a friend with whom to eat healthfully and work out. Significant others can be food pushers or saboteurs on cruises, saying things like, "We're on vacation, you can start again when we get back . . ." If you think you might have this problem, talk it through with your significant other *before* you go on the trip. Tell him or her how you'd like to handle the dinners and activities (for example, order the light fare, take fitness classes, and walk on the deck after dinner). Don't pressure or force your partner to do anything he or she doesn't want to do for your sake, but if your partner isn't on board with your plan (no pun intended), lay some ground rules—for example, ask him or her to agree *not* to

- Tempt you by offering you a bite of his or her food at meals

- Order room service after a certain time of night or while you're in the room

- Convince you to give up an activity in order to be his or her lounge lizard companion

• Buy you any food-related gifts

• Order anything for you or order something to share before talking it over with you

Working these issues out ahead of time can prevent you from ruining your vacation with one food fight after another!

Understand how true weight gain works—and doesn't. Many of Sass's clients tell her they went on a cruise and gained 10 pounds. However, in order to have gained 10 pounds of true body fat, you must eat the number of calories it takes to keep you at your current weight (usually 1,500 to 2,000) plus an additional 35,000 calories you did not burn off (1 pound of fat = 3,500 calories). That's a *lot* of eating. On a one-week cruise you'd have to *overeat* by 5,000 calories each day (i.e., your usual 2,000 plus 5,000 more, for a daily total of 7,000) to gain 10 pounds of true body fat. It's possible, but unlikely. The extra weight gain is often water weight. Just 2 cups of retained water causes your weight on the scale to go up by 1 pound. This vacation-induced water retention will eventually go away, however, when you get back to your usual environment and routine.

Don't starve yourself before you go on the cruise. Many people ask whether they should eat just one meal a day before going on the cruise if they know they'll be overeating on the cruise. The answer is NO! That is, in fact, the best way to gain weight. Cutting your calorie intake too far below what it takes to maintain your current weight sends your body into starvation mode. The result is that, while you're undereating, your body burns fewer calories per day to conserve energy, then on the cruise, when you're overindulging, you'll be storing fat like crazy due to your slower metabolism.

The following chart offers some notes and suggestions about eating healthy and staying fit, correlated to each cruise line.

	Royal Caribbean	Norwegian	Princess	Crystal	Celebrity	Carnival	Holland America
Overall Positives	Good variety of healthy food options; good variety of fitness options.	Good variety of healthy food options; good variety of fitness options. Calorie and nutrition facts provided for Cooking Light selections.	Some healthy food options available; good variety of fitness options.	Good variety of healthy food options; good variety of fitness options. Some of the nutrition and fitness information is provided by experts at the well-respected Cleveland Clinic.	Good variety of healthy food options; good variety of fitness options.	Good variety of healthy food options; good variety of fitness options. Calorie and nutrition facts provided for Spa selections.	Fair variety of healthy food options; good variety of fitness options.
Overall Negatives	No calorie or nutrition facts information on menus.	It could be difficult to resist the other menu items and meals on this cruise!	No calorie or nutrition facts information on menus; somewhat limited dining selections compared to, say, Norwegian.	Going with the low-carb menu can zap you of the energy and endurance you need to participate in physical activity. Some of the low-carb options could be quite high in cholesterol	No calorie or nutrition facts information on the menus. It could be difficult to resist the other menu items and meals on this cruise!	Going with the low-carb menu can zap you of the energy and endurance you need to participate in physical activity.	It could be *very difficult* to resist the other menu items and meals on this cruise! According to the information reviewed, "HA is long known for the most extensive menus at sea."

There is a free ice cream bar featuring all the trimmings to make your own sundaes, complimentary hot hors d'oeuvres during cocktail hour, 24-hour free room service, and the traditional late-night buffet, one of which is a Chocolate Extravaganza! In addition, there is no designated low-calorie or light menu or menu options and no calorie or nutrition fact information for the menus. If you're looking to pig out, this is the cruise for you.

and saturated fat. No calorie or nutrition facts information on the menus.

	Royal Caribbean	Norwegian	Princess	Crystal	Celebrity	Carnival	Holland America
Best Menu Choices	*Breakfast:* Whole grain cereal with skim milk, fresh fruit, and a side of scrambled eggs would be a great way to start the day. Avoid the hash browns, sausage, bacon, pastries, etc. *Meals:* The Royal Lifestyle meals denoted with a symbol on the menus are wonderful. Options include light salads and soups, roasted red pepper hummus, and grilled fish and	Anything from the Cooking Light options at Pacific Heights—just be sure to look at the calories. At Bamboo, stick with the Seared Ahi or Tofu and Vegetable Curry option and skip the rice if you want a bite of dessert. Avoid Cagney's and Le Bistro—the menus are very indulgent! At Salsa, stick with Chicken Fajitas (limit to two tortillas, watch your portions of cheese and	For room service, stick with the roast turkey sandwich on wheat, skip the fries, chips, and coleslaw, and have a mixed garden salad with low-calorie dressing. *Meals:* The spa menus are certainly filled with healthy ingredients but there is no calorie or nutrition facts information and many menus include creamy/fatty items such as cream soups,	The "On the Lighter Side" options are great, but there are no calorie numbers provided. Options include grilled fish, pork medallions, and grilled chicken breast, but the desserts seem to be limited to sorbet or sherbet. You may be better off splitting a regular dessert and going for a walk or dancing after dinner.	Several special menus are available including "Lean and Light," vegetarian, diabetic, and low-fat. These will be your best bets. *Breakfast:* Choose whole grain hot or cold cereal with nuts or seeds added, and fresh fruit. Avoid muffins, pastries, and bagels. Be careful with the smoothies; some are made with added syrups and sugars or are so large that the calo-	The Spa selections are wonderful. They include options such as Pacific Salmon, Tiger Shrimp, Tomato Mozzarella Salad, and low-cal soups. Calorie and fat information is provided. Other good main course options (not Spa menu) include Catch of the Day, Vegetable Curry, and Smoked Turkey Tenderloin. Several salad and vegetable-based appetizers are also	*Breakfast:* In the Lido dining area there are healthy cereals, yogurt, fresh fruit, and cholesterol-free egg white omelets. These are your best bets if you can stay away from the muffins and pastries. There are fat-free muffins but avoid these— they are very high in calories and loaded with sugar. A small serving of whole grain cereal with either skim milk or yogurt

mixed into it, a small egg white omelet with veggies (no cheese), and a small side of fresh fruit would be an ideal breakfast. Every dinner menu has either seafood, chicken, or both entrées available. However, they are accompanied by rich sauces and side dishes such as plantains, creamed potatoes, and saffron risotto cakes. Order chicken, fish, or any tenderloin dinner but ask for any sauce on the side so you can control

available such as Grilled Baby Vegetables, Tomato Artichoke Salad, and Chilled Zucchini Soup. Only the Spa menu lists calories, however.

rie levels are several hundred, yet they aren't filling. For the AquaSpa Café, stick with the "Light Fare" options, which include items such as poached salmon, vegetable sushi, and roast turkey breast. Stateroom Service offers veggie burgers and wraps, and grilled chicken and smoked salmon sandwiches. At the Olympic restaurant, stick with broth-based soups, salads with low-cal dressing, and

fettuccine Alfredo, mashed potatoes, and french fries. Stick with grilled or baked seafood and chicken entrées, broth-based soups, and salads with light dressings. The bottom of the menu states that you can ask for modifications for special dietary needs, so don't be afraid to ask for things without butter or sauces, smaller portions, etc.

sour cream, and use salsa generously) or the Blackened Mahimahi.

chicken entrées. *Dessert:* Low-fat and sugar-free options are available, but these aren't always low in calories and may not be satisfying. You may be better off splitting a regular dessert and going for a walk or out dancing after dinner.

	Royal Caribbean	Norwegian	Princess	Crystal	Celebrity	Carnival	Holland America
					grilled or baked seafood options. At the Metropolitan, stick with roasted chicken, broiled tilapia, cod, snapper, or lean tenderloin options but sub grilled veggies or a dinner salad for the mashed potatoes.		how much you use, and ask for a sub of steamed or grilled veggies instead of the heavier starch-based sides.
Other Menu Notes	Avoid the selections labeled "Light Meals." Assume the word "light" here refers to the size of the meals because	No breakfast information.	No breakfast information.	No breakfast information.	No additional notes.	No breakfast information.	Vegetarian meals can be ordered 24 hours in advance — these aren't always low-cal, and many are made with

the selections are not light on calories or fat. Options include burgers, and salads topped with fatty cheeses, croutons, eggs, and dressings. It's also not clear if the cottage cheese and yogurt are low-fat. If you must order from this menu, stick with a turkey sandwich with cheese but skip the potato chips it comes with and ask to get it on whole wheat bread instead of French.

cheeses and cream sauces. A few no-sugar-added desserts are available, but there is no calorie or nutrition facts information to compare to the other desserts, and since these tend to be unsatisfying, you may wind up eating the real thing anyway, or overeating the no-sugar-added desserts. Fortunately, there are great fitness options on this cruise so if you have the breakfast described, and stick with fish or grilled

	Royal Caribbean	Norwegian	Princess	Crystal	Celebrity	Carnival	Holland America
							chicken with veggies for dinner, you can afford to have a few bites of a decadent dessert if you're active after dinner. Overall, however, this cruise line requires willpower!
Fitness Notes	Great selection of fitness equipment including twenty treadmills, and other aerobic and strength training machines.	Equipment wasn't listed by name but a twenty-four-hour fitness center is available as well as spinning, aerobics, yoga, Pilates, yoga, pools, and basketball courts.	Great selection of fitness equipment including seventeen treadmills, other aerobic and strength training machines, and numerous classes including dancing, power walk-	Great selection of fitness equipment including eight to ten treadmills, other aerobic and strength training machines, and numerous classes including Pilates, yoga, body sculpting, and	Equipment wasn't listed completely, but a well-stocked fitness center is available as well as classes including spinning, yoga, Pilates, kickboxing, and personal training (at some cost extra).	Equipment wasn't listed completely, but there is a 13,300-square-foot spa and fitness center including treadmills, stair climbers, bikes, free weights, and group fitness classes such	One great thing about HA is the Fitness Fanatics Guide to Cruising. It maps out a fitness plan for each of the eight days and provides the number of calories that would be burned (this

as spinning, yoga, and kickboxing.		varies based on weight, and they didn't provide the weight they used to calculate these, so if you're a 5-foot, 2-inch female who weighs 125 pounds, the calorie burning may be overestimated for you—you'll probably burn less than what these numbers say, which could lead you to eat too much if you think you're burning more than you are). There is also a well-stocked fitness center with treadmills and stair steppers in front of the windows
	circuit training.	
ing, and kickboxing (some are at additional cost).		

	Royal Caribbean	Norwegian	Princess	Crystal	Celebrity	Carnival	Holland America
							facing the view. Group fitness classes are offered daily including yoga, Pilates, and water-based classes, but there is an additional fee for these. There are also volleyball and tennis courts.

Lap Calc

On the track, 5 laps = 1 mile.	*Jewel:* 2.5 laps = 1 mile. *Star* and *Dawn:* 3.5 laps = 1 mile.	On Grand-class ships, 3 times around the promenade deck, or 10 laps around the jogging track = 1 mile.	On *Symphony,* 3.7 laps around ship = 1 mile. On *Serenity,* 3.35 laps = 1 mile.	No information available.	On all ships, 8 laps around the jogging track = 1 mile.	For *Amsterdam* and *Volendam,* 3.5 laps on promenade = 1 mile. *Maasdam, Statendam,* and *Zaandam:* 4 on lower promenade = 1 mile. *Noordam, Oosterdam,* and *Zuiderdam:* 3 laps on promenade = 1 mile. *Prinsendam,* 4.5 laps on promenade = 1 mile.

GET MOVING

Remember the old image of a cruise passenger, sitting in a deck chair, doing nothing but eating finger sandwiches and drinking? Now it's time to get off that chair and start moving. In my case, that meant going to the *Summit*'s fitness center.

The opportunities to exercise on board have become more attractive. Like those at hotels, cruise ship fitness centers are no longer the cold little rooms in the depths of the ship. Today, many ships boast fitness centers as luxurious as the captain's quarters, and they occupy prime locations—often perched on the top decks with great views. And the activities themselves have become more diverse. Royal Caribbean features an on-board climbing wall; Princess Cruises started the Lotus Spa & Fitness Program, offering yoga and Pilates classes as well as kickboxing and spinning; and Crystal Cruises even offers cruisers a complete itinerary dedicated to health and fitness.

The trend toward fitness may be due in part to an evolving clientele. Cruise demographics are changing. "No longer the newlywed and nearly dead," says Major. "The average age today is fifty." A younger, health-and-fitness-minded clientele has pushed ships to go that extra mile on and off the ship.

And no, walking around the deck two times does not entitle you to that piece of cheesecake at the end of the meal. Not even close. I did some checking (and some walking, too), and here are the real figures:

- *Celebrity and Royal Caribbean:* The average track takes five laps to complete 1 mile, which means that one lap equals $2/10$ of a mile.

- *Crystal:* 3.7 laps equals 1 mile.

- *Celebrity:* On my cruise, I attempted to do twenty laps of the ship each morning, totaling 4 miles.

Another thing cruise ships have in common with hotels: Fitness centers in both have pathetically low utilization rates. In fact, the rates for many cruise ships are even worse than those for hotels. Almost without exception, every time I went to the ship's fitness center, the only other people there (besides myself and the trainer) were dancers and gymnasts who were entertainers on the ship!

As for myself, there wasn't a day on my cruise that I didn't hit the fitness center. Again, I followed the same regimen provided by Annette Lang, working with the ship's trainer, Josh Thurbon. We modified it, of course, using more exercise balls, which made things interesting when the ship pitched and rolled. But we survived.

"Being on a ship can actually be an advantage," Thurbon told me. "The gym travels with you. You don't have to drive to get there, fight traffic. You just go up a few flights of stairs to one of the top decks and here we are." He had a point. Another advantage on a ship: You can always skip the elevators and take the stairs between decks. On some ships, like the *Queen Mary 2*, there can be as many as nineteen decks!

Thurbon put me through daily one-hour routines, but he is convinced that a thirty-minute-a-day program is enough to save just about anyone from the 8-pound curse.

On my cruise, only six other people worked with Josh and the other trainers on board—the participation numbers were that low. What that means is that if you plan properly for your cruise, you may have to wait for that massage or manicure, but you won't have to wait for a trainer. And that also means . . . no excuses.

The other good news is that almost every cruise ship I have visited has upgraded its fitness facilities. In some cases, cruise lines have dedicated 20,000 square feet of space to their fitness centers, with a full complement of resistance machines and free weights, plus cardiovascular equipment and the latest in health and fitness classes including Pilates, tai chi, yoga, and step aerobics.

EXERCISE ON BOARD

Here is a rundown, cruise line by cruise line, of the fitness options available to you when you travel by sea.

Carnival Cruise Lines

The Spa Carnival program on Carnival cruise ships offers guests the latest workout equipment and sessions for aerobics, relaxation, and stretching; as well as a range of European-style spa therapies, in spacious quarters on board. For diet watchers, Carnival Spa Fare provides cuisine that is lower in fat, sodium, cholesterol, and calories than typical cruise-line meals.

Celebrity Cruises

The AquaSpas on Celebrity's cruise ships feature state-of-the-art fitness centers where guests can work with free weights, advanced weight-training machines, and cardiovascular exercise equipment, as well as utilizing the aerobics areas. Trainers are available for personal instruction. A bonus is the panoramic vistas designed for each spa. Holistic spa treatments, massage rooms, saunas, steam rooms, thalassotherapy pools, and fully equipped beauty salons are among the other highlights. Many of the line's ships also feature AquaSpa Cafés, which offer healthful cuisine for every meal.

Costa Cruises

On Costa Cruises' ships you can take Pilates and yoga classes, among others, and indulge yourself by choosing from a comprehensive spa menu of massages and beauty treatments. The main dining rooms feature Health & Well-Being selections. The line's new ship, the *Costa Concordia*, includes the innovative two-deck Samsara Spa, which guests can access via a private elevator from the fifty-five cabins and twelve suites on board.

Crystal Cruises

Crystal Cruises ships' spas are the only ones at sea that have been designed using feng shui principles. Several health and fitness theme cruises are scheduled annually, and each focuses on a different program such as Pilates, tai chi, or yoga. Fitness centers offer a roster of classes that changes every day. At mealtimes, diners can choose from the three-course, low-carbohydrate menus, opting from selections that are low in salt, fat, sugar, and cholesterol, according to their dietary needs.

Cunard Line

The Cunard Line's flagship *Queen Mary 2* features a Canyon Ranch SpaClub on board, with 20,000 square feet of dedicated facilities on two decks. This is the first Canyon Ranch facility on a luxury liner, and to complete the experience, Canyon Ranch chefs prepare the spa dishes that are served in the *QM2* dining rooms.

Disney Cruise Line

The *Disney Magic*'s Vista Spa & Salon features "spa villas" consisting of three indoor/outdoor treatment suites, each including a private verandah with a hot tub, an open-air shower, and a chaise lounge. The fitness center has been expanded to accommodate additional cardiovascular and weight machines and more space for the aerobics, yoga, and body shaping classes offered there.

Holland America Line

You can select from a comprehensive menu of massage and body treatments, facials, detoxification therapies, and salon services for men and women offered by Holland America's Greenhouse Spas. At the fitness centers, you can work out using top-of-the-line weight and cardio machines or take classes in Pilates, yoga, or spinning. Lunch and dinner menus feature healthy selections in the main dining rooms and Lido buffets.

MSC Cruises

You can pamper yourself with a wide variety of spa treatments if you cruise with MSC. The MSC ships *Opera, Lirica, Sinfonia,* and *Armonia* each have relaxation and meditation rooms, in addition to fitness centers and beauty salons. You can choose from classes in yoga, Pilates, and aerobics. Lunch and dinner menus offer "Healthy Choice" and vegetarian dishes, and also make sugar-free desserts available.

Norwegian Cruise Line

The Mandara Spas on Norwegian Cruise Line and NCL America ships feature such treatments as hot stone massages, Hawaiian Lomi Lomi massages, Swedish-style massage, and reflexology. There are twenty-four-hour fitness centers, jogging tracks, and volleyball and basketball courts, as well as putting greens, steam rooms, fitness classes, and gyms with cardio equipment, weight machines, and free weights available to guests.

Oceania Cruises

Mandara Spas also operates the facilities for Oceania Cruises, where you will find thalassotherapy whirlpools and spa cabanas for on-deck massages. You can sign up for yoga and Pilates classes or work with a personal trainer provided by the cruise line. Visit one of the styling salons for hairstyling, facials, manicures, and pedicures. Dining rooms feature Oceania Spa Cuisine, and guests dining in Toscana and the Polo Grill can request light and healthy cuisine.

Princess Cruises

Enjoy an Asian-themed atmosphere and treatments based on Far Eastern therapies and rituals including facials, body treatments, and massages, at the Lotus Spas on Princess Cruises ships. In addition, you can take exercise classes, work with a fitness instructor, or request personal training and consultation sessions. A series of health and nutrition seminars are also available.

Radisson Seven Seas Cruises

The "spotlight" cruises offered by Radisson Seven Seas Cruises feature lectures by experts on the benefits of staying active and eating a healthy diet. At the Carita Spas, guests can treat themselves to the dry saunas, steam baths, and Jacuzzis. The ships feature fully equipped gyms, and classes in aerobics, step aerobics, stretching, and body toning are available. In the dining rooms, you can choose from a menu of lean and healthy entrées.

Royal Caribbean International

At Royal Caribbean's onboard ShipShape Fitness Centers, guests can choose from a wide range of options including cardiovascular equipment, weight machines, and stair steppers; yoga, kickboxing, and aerobics classes and personal training sessions; and jogging tracks, basketball courts, rock-climbing walls, miniature golf, and golf simulators. The ShipShape Spas likewise feature a variety of unique treatments, including Elemis Aroma Stone Therapy, Swedish massage, hydralift facials, and enriching milk baths.

Seabourn Cruise Line

The 2005 *Condé Nast Traveler* Readers' Survey awarded the highest score for an onboard spa to The Spa at Seabourn, which has full-service facilities on each of the three all-suite *Yachts of Seabourn*. Guests can choose from such featured delights as Elemis Aroma Stone Therapy, LT Oxygen Lifting Facials, and

Aroma Spa Ocean Wraps. To acquaint guests with the soothing nature of massage therapy, complimentary Massage Moments are offered on deck.

Silversea Cruises

Mandara Spas are again featured on all four of Silversea Cruises' ships. Guests can select from services including dry and steam saunas, beauty and hair salons, and fitness centers and classes including stretching, aerobics, Pilates, and yoga. Instruction in circuit training is available, and you can request one-on-one training sessions at an additional charge. The ships' dining rooms offer CruiseLite and low-carb menus.

Swan Hellenic

On board Swan Hellenic's *Minerva II,* guests are offered a range of treats, from Reiki and reflexology to manicures and makeup application. Fitness fanatics can choose from Pilates; yoga; tai chi; circuit class; body toning; Body Ball; Body Breathe; Body Stretch; Legs, Bums, and Tums; and the Walking Club, all of which are led by a fitness director or a certified personal trainer.

Windstar Cruises

Windstar Cruises' *Wind Star* and *Wind Spirit* feature expanded gyms with new equipment, to meet the fitness needs of the 148 passengers that each of these luxury liners can accommodate. The *Wind Surf*'s WindSpa likewise offers an updated gym, with a Nautilus room, additional fitness classes, and spa treatments that include everything from traditional massage and aromatherapy to hydrotherapy and synergistic therapy. All Windstar ships offer healthy meal choices and vegetarian selections in the dining rooms.

OK, so much for exercising on the ship. What about when the ship is in port? (About five out of every seven days at sea.)

EXERCISE ON SHORE

You can make your shore excursion an active one. You don't have to sit on a bus to see a museum or historic place. Excursions from cruise lines now include everything from ziplining across Costa Rican rain forests to rock climbing.

And never underestimate the benefits of just . . . walking!

In the meantime, here are some of the more physically active shore excursions offered by cruise lines.

Celebrity Xpeditions

While your ship is docked in Hamilton, Bermuda, you can take a seven-hour water excursion aboard a catamaran to Blue Cur Barrier Reef, where the captain will brief you on the lore of the area, including the tale of a shipwreck. Guests can snorkel over the wreck. Price: $650.

A considerably more affordable adventure is the St. George's Kayak Safari. It's just you and the fish during this two-hour paddling tour in a glass-bottom kayak. Price: $64. (www.celebrity.com)

Crystal Cruises

If *Splash* is your favorite movie and you still have dreams about being the Little Mermaid, you can almost make that dream a reality as you walk under the sea in Bora-Bora. On this expedition, passengers stroll beneath the crashing waves wearing a special diving helmet. Price: $73.

Your friends call you Skipper and your mother tells everyone you were born wearing deck shoes. Now, in St. Maarten you can learn how to race the crème de la crème—America's Cup retired yachts. Price: $75. (www.crystalcruises.com)

Carnival Cruise Lines

Brave the white waters of Mexico as you paddle these river rapids near Acapulco. The 8-kilometer trip will test your strength and make you earn that picnic lunch. Price: $100 to $149.

Looking for a wild time? Passengers cruising to Alaska can go on an Alaskan Bear Adventure. Take a floatplane to the Tongass National Forest, where a naturalist will take you on a hike to a spot where you can watch bears feeding on salmon. Price: $150+. (www.carnival.com)

Holland America

After floating at a leisurely pace, you may feel the need for speed. Cruisers stopping in Barcelona can visit the Formula 1 circuit in Montmelo, then ride their own 270-cc, four-cylinder go-carts on a separate track. Price: $138.

If you are cruising the North American East Coast looking for a revolutionary experience, consider enlisting as a "soldier for a day." In Halifax, Nova Scotia, the Halifax Citadel will dress you up in kilt and bonnet and teach you how to use the weaponry of the infamous Redcoats. Price: $299. (www.holland america.com)

Norwegian Cruise Line

Say aloha to one of Hawaii's tallest peaks. You won't have to climb up—just race 38 miles down Mount Haleakala. You won't have to pedal too much on this eight-hour cycling tour—that's a promise. Price: $149.

If whizzing through the trees is more your speed, Kauai cruisers can take a three-and-a-half hour Canopy Zip Line tour through the sweet-smelling Kauaian vegetation. Price: $149. (www.ncl.com)

Silversea Cruises

If remote locations are more to your liking, take a trip to the final frontier—Antarctica. Cruisers on the Fire and Ice trip to southern South America can hop a plane to Antarctica, where they can tour a Chilean research station and march with the penguins. Price: $2,995.

Perhaps even more exotic than a trip to the icy south is a journey to the cold war capital via fighter jet. Cruise passengers to Northern Europe and the Baltic area can take a one-day excursion to Moscow, flying on a MIG fighter jet to get there. Price: a mere $13,000. (www.silversea.com)

Princess Cruises

Take in the Greek island of Santorini by sea and land. Princess's Sailing and Hiking Expedition takes passengers for a hike up the Santorini volcano, where you get an excellent view of the island. Price: $39.

Pining for the fjords? Don't pine—paddle. Passengers cruising through Norway can kayak the Aurlandfjord. Paddle past tranquil farmland and grazing sheep, and imagine the Norway of yesteryear. Price: $74. (www.princess.com)

If you don't want to feel limited to booking shore excursions through your cruise line, independent shore excursion companies offer passengers alternatives to cruise-ship-organized excursions and help you venture beyond the bow of your ship.

Shore Trips

Hike through the Costa Rican rain forest with a guide who can point out the flora and fauna that you meet along the way. Price: $81 per person.

Julie Ansfield and Barry Karp offer over 2,200 shore excursion options, from the Mediterranean to the Caribbean. Participants are guaranteed on-time arrival back to the ship or their money back. (www.shoretrips.com)

Port Compass

This independent shore excursion company offers cruisers another alternative to ship-planned and -priced excursions around Europe and the Americas. Trek up a Hawaiian volcano on the Kilauea Volcano Discovery Hike, a 14-mile trek along the Big Island's most active volcano. Price: $135 per person. (www.portcompass.com)

Aloha Top Ten

Swim with the sandbar and grayreef sharks in Oahu on the two-hour North Shore Adventure, which costs $125 per person. For more information about this and other Hawaiian day excursions, go to http://alohatopten.com.

Port Promotions

Port Promotions guarantees shore excursions at discounted prices without making you wait in long cruise-ship lines. Passengers can choose prepackaged trips such as the Mush the Yukon Dogsled Experience in Alaska ($165 per person) and the Hike and Float Adventure down the Taiya River ($95 per person) in Alaska, or they can customize their own tours for large groups or a family looking for a more one-on-one experience. (www.portpromotions.com)

Shore Tours

This is one of my favorite websites—and it acts as a gateway for passengers to book independent shore activities directly from vendors. What this means is you can tailor your own shore excursions to just about any cruise-ship itinerary. Click on your port of call and Shore Tours will provide you with links to local tour and adventure providers such as a kayak and canoe outfitter in Ketchikan, Alaska, or a scuba diving outfit in Argentina. (www.shoretours.com)

And some final words of advice . . .

Don't catch a virus! It's not the preferred weight loss method.

The VSP (Vessel Sanitation Program) of the Centers for Disease Control and Prevention in Atlanta oversees sanitation conditions on cruise ships. Inspectors from the VSP inspect each ship twice a year by showing up without warning when the ship arrives at a port.

Cruise ships are subject to a forty-two-item checklist on a rating system. Most violations cost one to five points. Anything over eighty-six points is considered a pass; below eighty-six is failing. Luckily, you now have access to the VSP's "green sheet," where you can check how your prospective ship rates on the cleanliness scale. VSP sanitation scores and reports for specific ships are available at www.cdc.gov/nceh/vsp.

Because cruise ships are, by definition, operating within close quarters, the CDC recommends that you be up to date with immunizations, especially flu shots; that you get the recommended immunizations for the countries you are visiting; and that you pay particular attention to hand hygiene, either by washing with soap and water or by using an alcohol-based hand sanitizer. As a further health measure, cruise-ship spas must be drained and sanitized every night.

But here's the best news of all: I disembarked the *Summit* weighing a half pound *less* than when I boarded. Not a staggering loss, but considering it was a cruise, this is really Victory at Sea.

CHAPTER 9

Jet Lag, Sleep, and Weight: What You Need to Know

OK, please don't hate me . . . but I don't get jet lag. To the best of my recollection, I never have been afflicted with it. There are those medical experts who would disagree with me. But more on that later.

Then there's the issue of sleep itself. No matter how much you talk about diet, exercise, fitness, food, and travel, the great imponderable has always been sleep—how much we need, how much we get, and how it affects our performance, both physical and mental, especially when we travel. And now, new research indicates a direct link between sleep, or lack of it, and weight gain. This is of major interest to travelers—and obviously, to me.

I've already discussed what I eat—or more accurately—don't eat when flying. But I have another strategy that I suspect also helps keep the weight down: I do not take any medications to help me sleep, or help me fly, or help me avoid jet lag. My flying philosophy is really quite simple. If I'm awake and want to read on the flight, I read. If I want to work, I work. If I want to slip into a light coma, I'll do that as well. But for me, it's not what you do on the plane, it's what you do when you land that counts—and that often makes the difference between a severe bout of extended jet lag and, as in my case, no jet lag whatsoever.

After a long flight—no matter when the plane lands—I force myself to stay awake until at least 11 P.M. local time. And I will do *anything* not to sleep when I arrive. I'll take a walk; I'll shoot hoops; I might take a shower in the middle of the afternoon. Anything. If I succumb to that temptation of the 4 P.M. "little nap," I won't wake up for at least three days, and when I do, I won't remember my name. So I will do whatever is necessary to stay awake throughout that first arrival day. And then I hit the sack around 11 P.M. or midnight.

I don't totally cycle the first night. I generally get about three hours' sleep. But the next night is perfect: I'll do my normal four-and-a-half hours.

And yet, so many of my friends—and I presume many of your friends, perhaps even you—get jet lag from flying on the shuttle between New York and LaGuardia or between Los Angeles and San Francisco. For these people, just the thought of an airplane flight makes jet lag kick in. They become jet lag victims, suffering from sluggishness, fatigue, lack of appetite, disorientation, lack of concentration, and lightheadedness. And it can actually take their bodies a full day to recover from each time zone crossed. (Which is why I can't understand why jet lag would happen when someone travels within the same time zone. The culprit must be . . . stress!)

Everyone, it seems, has a theory about how best to conquer jet lag: melatonin, Ambien, Lunesta, Sonata . . . then there's light therapy, caffeine, walking—and yes, even sleeping. I know folks—and I'm not kidding—whose remedy for jet lag is to go bowling at midnight! And as I've come to learn, if you don't understand jet lag and sleep on the road, you are going to gain weight.

I'm one of those diehards who believe that jet lag is simply a state of mind. But before we get to my theories, let's first look at a medical approach to dealing with jet lag.

Our circadian rhythms support maximum alertness and energy efficiency during the day, and promote rest and rejuvenation during sleep. After flying over multiple time zones, we're displaced in time. At the destination, the twenty-four-hour cycle of environmental and social demands on the body is much different than at home, and our biological time structure is unsynchronized and scrambled. So if you believe that the human body is a machine that runs—almost literally—like clockwork, then you might assume you are doomed every time you travel.

Of course, the health and beauty industry wants us to believe that the solution to this problem is aromatherapy, or a hot bath, or a great bed. Or a pill.

Not even close, according to most scientists. They insist that jet lag is not simply a mental condition. Of course, dehydration, high altitudes, and stress might contribute to jet lag. But they do not cause it. Scientists argue that jet lag is first and foremost a physical condition, and this condition is worsened by high altitudes, dry air, and stress. Jet lag is simply a result of all our biological clocks being broken at the same time.

So is it merely a matter of how much sleep you can get and when you can get it? Not quite. Jet lag is really the result of being *sleep deprived.* One of the things that happens to airplane travelers is that they become sleep deprived because the flight is too short. Couple that with their sleep patterns on the ground, and you have a full-tilt recipe for jet lag. Over the last fifty years, Americans have pared about two hours from their nightly sleep times. About 40 percent of adults get less than seven hours of sleep each night.

Now, let's put that in the context of a plane flight. In the 1950s, a flight from New York to Europe averaged about fifteen hours—time for dinner, conversation with friends, and . . . sleep (and in those days, the planes had berths!). Today, an overnight journey through the same five time zones leaves barely enough time to watch the movie and eat that terrible airline meal.

Add to that the concept of losing time. That eastbound flight with a night departure—from New York to, let's say, Paris—may last seven hours. But that's not all air time. Air time amounts to about six hours, and of that time, the first thirty minutes is spent gaining altitude. Then the flight attendants serve a beverage, followed by a meal, which can take an hour. That leaves only four-and-a-half hours to sleep. But even that is eroded by the last thirty minutes of the flight, during descent, when you have to sit upright and fill out your customs and immigration forms. So you have roughly three-and-a-half hours of potential sleep time—and that assumes no interruptions.

To complicate the situation, there's the issue of the real clock versus your internal clock. When you leave New York, your body thinks it's 9:30 P.M., and that's because it *is* 9:30 P.M. But when you land seven hours later, your body thinks it's 4:30 A.M. when it's actually 10:30 A.M. in Paris. And that, of course, explains why your head droops to your stomach in the middle of that meeting later the same day.

Even worse is when you get on a super-long-haul flight, such as the eighteen-hour nonstop between New York and Singapore. That's when you might as well take your body clock—and the real clock—and throw them both out.

SNOOZE . . . YOU WIN

My advice, expecially on night flights: Instruct the flight attendants not to disturb you for the meal service, bring your own bottles of water, and go to sleep as soon as you possibly can after takeoff.

Another factor in the sleep equation is the air quality and temperature in the cabin. I am convinced they affect your ability to sleep—or sleep better.

Remember, the higher the altitude, the greater the sleep disruption. If you're flying higher than 13,200 feet (and trust me, you will be), diminished oxygen levels and changes in your own respiration will combine to mess you up. The point at which sleep is disturbed is also a function of temperature. Temperatures above 75°F or below 54°F will definitely wake you up.

Cabin air is a mix of fresh air, brought in from outside the plane, and filtered, recirculated air. In addition, it's drier than the Sahara. Here's a scary thought: One piece of research published in *Anaesthesia*, the official journal of the Association of Anaesthetists of Great Britain (one of the few magazines I don't get regularly) indicates that more than half of airline passengers are starved for quality air—oxygen—at high altitudes. For 54 percent of air travelers, the drop in oxygen level at a high altitude was at least 6 percent. Translation: If you were a hospital patient, the nurses would be calling for . . . more oxygen! The solution here is also a simple one: When boarding the plane, ask the flight attendants to request that the cockpit crew activate all three air pacs on board. If they do, you stand a better chance of getting more oxygen in flight.

Whether lack of sufficient oxygen is the culprit or not, a recent British Airways survey found that on flights between New York and London, the average economy-class passenger gets only three hours of sleep. Even if you spring for business class, you're likely to get only four hours. This doesn't bode well for people who are expected to perform on the job the next day. The British Airways research revealed that of one thousand people surveyed, 25 percent admitted to falling asleep in a meeting following a flight, and nearly one in five claimed their business meeting or presentation went badly as a result of poor sleep due to air travel.

This hasn't stopped the airlines from trying to go back to the future—devising "new" lie-flat beds for business class and, on some ultra-long-haul flights, installing coach seats that recline more comfortably. The research showed that airplane travelers who occupied seat beds got an average of an hour more sleep than coach fliers.

WHEN YOU ARRIVE

A lot of experts suggest that to help combat jet lag, you should set your watch to the time zone of your destination. I never do this. I'm more interested in what everyone back home is doing. If I want to know what time it is in my new locale, I can look at the clock in my hotel room. Instead, my anti–jet lag strategy is to just go for a walk. If your plane arrives in the morning, expose yourself to sunlight, which will help reset your body clock. And take my advice: Do anything to prevent yourself from taking a long nap as soon as you arrive.

Dr. Timothy Monk, a sleep expert at the University of Pittsburgh, recommends that you get daylight and exercise together in the morning before breakfast. That sends a message to your biological clock that morning has started. However, he advises travelers to minimize their evening light exposure. Try to nudge the clock in only one direction. "After 6 P.M., stay away from daylight. And recognize your sleep is going to be fragile," Dr. Monk counsels.

If you are flying west from Europe, rather than maximizing morning exposure, stay indoors and enhance evening light exposure. Take a brisk walk or jog just before sunset. Finally, Monk suggests, "When in Rome, do what the Romans do. Your meals and bedtimes should be scheduled according to local time unless you're there for twenty-four hours."

What dietary approaches can you take to treat jet lag? Dr. Monk has these suggestions: "Just to keep things simple, think of protein as something that's going to wake you up and carbs as something that make you sleepy. If you want to be woken up, you want to load up on proteins for breakfast; conversely, when you are trying to go to bed, then you want to be thinking about carbohydrates." Qualifying this, Dr. Monk continues, "Superceding that advice is to remember that you shouldn't be eating foods that are hard to digest. Common sense says that if you are going to have a spicy dish or a heavy pizza just before bedtime, this is a bad idea."

AT THE HOTEL

But the key component remains . . . sleep. The hotel business is always trying to improve it—or perhaps even reinvent it.

Hotels have studied road warriors like me for years, and for obvious reasons. They want to identify the links between great sleep and happy customers—if you get a good night's sleep at a hotel, you're more likely to return. Consider this 1999 study of travelers' sleeping habits, which seems to indicate that great sleep beats even great sex (*Sleeping on the Road,* a study by Westin Hotels & Resorts). Of the travelers surveyed, 63 percent said that a good night's sleep is the most important service a hotel can provide. Sleep is so important that more than twice as many travelers said they'd take a great night's sleep than opted for great sex (I'm serious!). Here are some other findings:

- Travelers said they get less sleep on the road as compared with home (49 percent), sleep fewer hours (51 percent), and are more likely to wake up in the middle of the night in a hotel bed (31 percent).

- The quality of sleep travelers get on the road is worse (50 percent), and 31 percent claim their performance on the road has suffered because of a bad night's sleep in a hotel room.

- Three-quarters of the executives surveyed said they're tired when they return home from a business trip and need to catch up on their sleep.

- On average, it takes a traveler twenty-four minutes to fall asleep in a hotel room, compared to fiftcen minutes at home.

Although that survey was done more than seven years ago, nothing much has changed in the intervening years.

Starwood used those survey results to justify installing 52,000 Heavenly Beds in its 39,500 guest rooms. These beds were certainly a welcome addition—they're plush, with custom-designed pillowtop mattresses, cozy down blankets, and three crisp, high-thread-count sheets on each one. But were the beds necessary? Of course they were. In that same Westin survey, women reported that if they were tossing and turning in their hotel bed, they were more likely to miss their own bed than the man they'd left behind (ouch).

Still, the beds didn't solve the jet lag problem. They didn't have a marked impact on the sleep deprivation of travelers, and they didn't stop frequent travelers from gaining weight on the road.

As the survey results suggested, sleeping well on the road is a more elusive concept for women than for men:

- It takes 54 percent of women more time to fall asleep in a hotel than at home, versus 35 percent of men.

- The quality of sleep in a hotel is worse than at home for 59 percent of women versus 47 percent of men.

- Women are much more likely to return home from a business trip tired (82 percent) than men (70 percent).

- When asked what they miss most about sleeping at home when they are sleeping in a hotel, their spouse or significant other is mentioned by 43 percent of men compared to only 22 percent of women.

  So what do women miss most when they're sleeping on the road? Their own bed (37 percent versus 22 percent of men). And while 66 percent of men say they'd like to bring their spouse or significant other along on a business trip, only 52 percent of women said the same.

- More women (93 percent) than men (81 percent) say a luxury bed makes a hotel room more attractive.

- When it comes to wardrobe in the boudoir, women are much more buttoned up than men. While 11 percent of men sleep in the nude and 42 percent sleep in their underwear, only

2 percent of women shed it all in bed and 3 percent strip to their skivvies.

The survey revealed some other interesting tidbits:

- When asked what keeps them up at night, 73 percent of the travelers surveyed say they miss their spouse or significant other, and 59 percent say they worry about what is going on back at the office.

- Most travelers (51 percent) would rather sleep in a hotel bed than in a bed at their mother-in-law's house (12 percent).

- One in three travelers (33 percent) admits to having an alcoholic beverage to help them fall asleep on the road.

- Travelers do many other things to help them fall asleep in hotel rooms, including reading (53 percent), calling their family (47 percent), drawing the curtains or shutting the blinds (43 percent), and leaving the TV on (42 percent).

- If they wake up in the middle of the night, travelers are most likely to watch TV (30 percent) or read (23 percent) to help them fall back asleep.

- Executives who watch TV in their hotel beds are a pretty serious lot, with CNN (79 percent), national network news (59 percent), and local network news (51 percent) being their top tube picks.

- Perhaps because they depend on TV to put them to sleep, travelers are more likely to watch thunderstorms and filibusters than adult movies in their hotel beds—42 percent of them say they watch the Weather Channel in their hotel rooms, while 17 percent surf to C-Span, and only 11 percent admit to watching adult movies.

• Who tucks business travelers in at night? Most travelers say the last voice they hear before going to sleep in a hotel room is that of their spouse or significant other (46 percent). On a less romantic note, 18 percent of travelers say goodnight to the wake-up service operator and 6 percent to the hotel operator.

Taking their cue from Starwood and the Heavenly Bed, other hotels entered the sleep research fray. More recently, Hilton, in cooperation with the National Sleep Foundation, surveyed more than one thousand business travelers from Japan, Germany, the United Kingdom, and the United States to learn more about sleep as it relates to travel. According to Hilton's performance study, for which participants actually wore a wrist actigraph to monitor sleep and wake patterns, business travelers reported getting almost one hour more sleep on a trip than they actually obtained. And the worst night of sleep was the night before departure—when travelers average only five hours of sleep. This study also found that participants' alcohol use increased 40 percent during the trip and their caffeine use increased 15 percent. Nearly half the travelers reported nodding off on a business trip, and here's something particularly frightening: Seventeen percent nodded off *while driving* after flying on a business trip.

The study also concluded that those who suffer from jet lag don't just eat at irregular times, but eat larger-than-normal-size portions. More than half of American and British business travelers surveyed eat more when they are away on business, and too many of them drink more when they are traveling. (The mistake here is that people think alcohol is a sleep inducer because it might initially make you feel drowsy or put you to sleep. In fact, it works to disrupt the most important, deeper levels of the sleep cycle.)

One of the more interesting results of this study was age-related, revealing an unexpected difference between road warriors and road rookies. "The picture of the aggressive young professional running circles around the older, weary business warrior does not apply when it comes to jet lag," the NSF survey reported. "In fact, the reverse appears to be true. Younger travelers (ages eighteen to forty-four) are nearly twice as likely (66 percent versus 36 percent) to '*not* feel as good as they would like during a business trip' as the older (45-years-old or older) travel-savvy veterans." Younger travelers also seem to have more trouble staying focused during business meetings when on the road than their older counterparts—they are almost twice as likely to be plagued by lack of focus (27 percent versus 15 percent). "This suggests an interesting, but unconfirmed, conclusion," contends the NSF survey. "The longer one travels, the better one may be able to cope with the effects of jet lag or other travel-related sleep disorders."

However, just when I thought there was hope for me, I encountered the much scarier topic of . . . sleep debt. "The bad news," says Dr. Mark Rosekind, former head of the Fatigue Countermeasures Program for NASA (now *there's* a job title), "is that when you lose sleep, it doesn't just disappear, but you actually build up a sleep debt." If that's true, then I filed Chapter 7 sleep bankruptcy about twenty years ago!

THE ARGUMENT FOR THE POWER NAP

Looks like I'll never be able to repay that sleep debt, but I can try to control it by taking power naps. Famous power nappers include Albert Einstein, Thomas Edison, Leonardo da Vinci, and Bill Clinton, so I know I'm in good company. But there's also a good scientific reason for it.

Dr. Rosekind studied NASA test pilots who were given planned, controlled forty-minute naps. The average pilot slept for twenty-six minutes—and performance improved 34 percent, while alertness was up 54 percent. Another good example of this phenomenon is the case of adventurer Steve Fossett. When he broke the record for nonstop, around-the-world solo flight in 2005, he did the nearly impossible—in sixty-seven hours of flight time, he slept only sixty minutes! And that sixty minutes was divided into a series of two- and three-minute high-flying power naps.

On a much less intense level, this is exactly what I do on the road, and as long as you practice full disclosure, you don't run the risk of folks thinking you're being rude or are a narcolepsy sufferer. On just about every trip I take, I already expect to be sleepless in Seattle, or New York, or London. Upon my arrival after a long flight, I tell my hosts that if we're driving, I plan to take ten-minute power naps en route, so they shouldn't think I'm ignoring them. On one trip to South Africa during which about eight separate meetings were scheduled for me each day, I took five- to seven-minute power naps in the car rides between meetings, and it all worked out fine. The most important nap every day: the ten-minute snooze I took just after lunch. I never napped more than fifteen minutes. If you make the nap too long, your body will think it's going into overnight sleep mode.

Sleep expert Dr. Martin Moore-Ede was a Harvard professor for twenty-five years and is now CEO of Circadian Technologies, an international research and consulting firm that helps companies with extended hours of operation. He says catnaps are a very effective way of sustaining energy. Naps of the ten-, fifteen-, or twenty-minute variety can be effective and constitute a good picker-upper. If you stick with naps that are short, you'll never get into the groggy state.

Dr. Moore-Ede also contends, however, that people have

different napability. You're either a morning type or an evening type. A long sleeper or a short sleeper. A napper or a consolidated sleeper. Flexible or rigid. Everyone is different.

SLEEPING MY WAY TO THE TOP

Successful power napping notwithstanding, I wanted to learn more about the conjunction of sleep, travel, and weight. I was still convinced that I don't suffer from jet lag, but if all the other research held true, then why hadn't I been able to lose weight on the road before I started the traveler's diet?

So I arranged to be fully examined at a sleep clinic. To be sure, most people who show up at a sleep clinic are there because they are among the nearly forty million Americans who suffer from one of eighty-four separate sleep disorders—the vast majority having insomnia. These are the folks who routinely struggle to get a good night's sleep. I, of course, was not one of them.

Heidi Skolnik got me an appointment at the Northern New Jersey Center for Sleep Medicine at Holy Name Hospital, in Teaneck, New Jersey. And my instructions were clear: I would arrive around 7 P.M. I was to bring pajamas or shorts, slippers and socks, and basic toiletries. That's it.

The moment I arrived, I would strip, and then be prepared for the polysomnogram (the overnight sleep study). Dr. John Villa, who runs the clinic, met me and explained the process. I would be fitted with thirty-two separate electrodes—on my head, chest, neck, legs, and back. This would take about ninety minutes. The electrodes would measure heart activity, brain wave activity, breathing, eye and leg movements, muscle tone, and blood oxygen levels. Infrared video cameras would record my physical movements throughout the night.

I was then led into my bedroom. It had a television, but no phone. And within ten minutes of my getting into bed—

gingerly, with all of those electrodes wired to my body—there was no television. It was lights-out.

The next morning, I was up at 5:30. It took about forty-five minutes to remove all the wires. And I returned to Manhattan. I felt I had slept well.

Less than a week later, the results were in. Remember, I'm the guy who insists I don't get jet lag. And every medical study insists that I *must* get jet lag, but that I may adjust better than others. Could this nonetheless negatively affect my diet? The answer is, sadly, yes.

First, the news about that polysomnogram.

"I have to tell you," Dr. Villa began, "that we really haven't seen anything like this."

Uh-oh . . .

But it seemed to be good news.

For starters, Dr. Villa reported something he referred to as most unusual: that I was exceptionally good at falling asleep in strange places. I told him I didn't find that surprising, since I sleep in strange places—hotel rooms—about three hundred nights a year. And so do most other road warriors. It's part of our inevitable ritual.

Still, Dr. Villa said that despite my being wired with dozens of electrodes, despite being in a strange room and knowing I would constantly be photographed, monitored, and taped, I actually fell asleep within three-and-a-half minutes of the lights being turned out in my room.

But wait. There was more. The clinic report also revealed that I had a "sleep efficiency" of 93.3 percent. Of the 357 minutes I was monitored, I slept for an astounding 333 minutes. And even better, I entered REM, or rapid eye movement, deep sleep in under an hour. Most people, Dr. Villa reports, take twice that long to get to that important sleep stage.

So that's excellent, right?

Not exactly. The most revealing statistics were yet to come. It wasn't that, as a frequent flier, I was able to get to sleep quickly and stay asleep consistently. The question Dr. Villa wanted answered: Was this the result of training myself to do this on a regular basis because of my routine, or was this the result of being sleep deprived?

"Let's dig a little deeper," Dr. Villa suggested. Then he hit me with the disturbing data. The Sleep Center staff recorded forty-three "respiratory events" during my sleep. "These respiratory events were repetitive and were associated with oxygen desaturation and marked disruption of sleep," they said. Specifically, I had stopped breathing forty-three times, the shortest for twenty-nine seconds and the longest for fifty-nine seconds!

What does that mean? A mild case of . . . sleep apnea.

Sleep apnea occurs when the soft tissue in the rear of your throat relaxes too much during sleep and partially blocks the passage, cutting off air. The result: loud snoring and labored breathing, until the breathing actually stops and the brain rouses you enough to gasp for air. Sure enough, the staff also recorded that during 13 percent of the time I slept, I snored! Dr. Villa explained that in many cases, sleep apnea is directly related to weight, and that the more weight I lost, the more the incidence of sleep apnea would most likely be reduced.

Then Dr. Villa told me the bad news: One of the reasons I fell asleep so quickly at the sleep center was not simply because I was a road warrior used to spending the night in strange environments, but because I was sleep deprived. In fact, he believed I was so chronically sleep deprived as a traveler that I no longer noticed how exhausted I really was.

But wait—it actually gets *worse.*

"Many frequent travelers," Villa reports, "are metabolic disasters. A frequent traveler with sleep deprivation is really bad. Plus, in many cases, that traveler will go after a high-carb diet in the morning. It's one big negative circle. We now live in a 24/7 world but our body just isn't designed for that."

And now, for the worst part of all: the link between sleep deprivation and weight gain. This is significant—not just in terms of the real rest I was receiving, but because of something perhaps more sinister: the way my brain was possibly sending out false signals of hunger.

And therein lies a big problem among travelers. Combine a rigorous travel schedule with sleep deprivation, and there's a direct correlation to obesity.

The truth is, scientists don't yet know the full biological effects of chronic sleep deprivation, but the picture doesn't look good. One of the most interesting lines of research is how sleep deprivation increases appetite.

Being overweight doesn't help sleeping, either. According to Dr. Charles Czeisler, head of Harvard Medical School's Division of Sleep Medicine at Brigham and Women's Hospital, older, obese men are at a higher risk for sleep apnea.

While some frequent travelers—like me—believe they function just fine on four hours of sleep, the medical establishment is almost unanimously in disagreement. In fact, they say not only might sleep deprivation be related to obesity, but it can impair job performance and increases the likelihood of automobile accidents. Ironically, one of the first things to go when we are sleep deprived is our cognitive ability to recognize how impaired we are.

Former NASA sleep expert Dr. Mark Rosekind says that sleep loss results in decreased memory function and impaired decision-making capacity. He says that memory functions decrease by 20 percent and decision-making capabilities can suffer by as much as 50 percent.

Dr. Czeisler says we are beginning to learn how important sleep is for performance. "One of the functions of sleep is the consolidation of memory," he explains. "If we go to a meeting to learn about some new process, where the memory of what we have learned is important, the night before is important so that we stay awake; the night after is important for consolidation of memory."

The problem, of course, is that we are fighting for sleep in a culture that doesn't value it—even among sleep experts. "I'm president of the sleep research society which is organizing a conference called Sleep 2006," says Dr. Czeisler. "They should call it No Sleep 2006, as they have scheduled events from seven in the morning to ten at night. And they're even talking about having something beforehand. This cultural imperative is so strong it's almost impossible to change where the ship is sailing."

Here's one thing Dr. Czeisler and his colleagues should perhaps add to their worries: If recent evidence is any indication, the folks leaving that conference are probably going to weigh more . . .

"People who are sleep deprived," says Dr. Meir Kryger, past president of the American Academy of Sleep Medicine, "actually get hungry." Basic translation: When you're tired, you're more likely to go on that dreaded Oreo patrol. A recent study by Eastern Virginia Medical School showed that people who reported getting eight hours of sleep (versus those with just over seven hours per night) had a body mass index (BMI) 5.5 points lower on average—the equivalent of 33 pounds *less*.

Things were beginning to make sense. This explained why my eating patterns were so crazy—why I felt the need to eat early, late, and . . . too often.

It's really about understanding two hormones—and false signals. Just ask Dr. Eve Van Cauter, who runs the Research Laboratory on Sleep, Chronobiology and Neuroendocrinology at the University of Chicago School of Medicine. She's spent more than twenty-five years doing research on the hormones that are affected by sleep.

"We are working on the issue of jet lag and sleep loss," she explains, "and all the evidence points to sleep loss as a risk factor for obesity. When we restrict sleep duration in healthy, lean, normal adults, we quickly observe two alterations. Leptin, the hormone that regulates appetite, the hormone that promotes satiety, the feeling of fullness, actually decreases." (When leptin levels are high, you feel satiated. If you're feeling hungry, leptin levels have dropped.) And that, coupled with increased levels of ghrelin, the hunger hormone, sends false signals to the brain when you're sleep deprived that you're starving, when, in fact, you're just the opposite. Hunger is increased even when your caloric intake has been more than sufficient.

"It's a double negative caused by sleep deprivation," Professor Van Cauter reports, "and the challenge for frequent travelers is to understand the false signals. Otherwise, short sleep is a direct risk factor for weight gain."

Specifically, short sleepers who are not natural short sleepers experience an alteration in which their body metabolizes glucose differently. If your sleep is artificially shortened, you need more insulin to metabolize and absorb the same amount of sugar—and you become a prime candidate for weight gain because your cravings for foods high in sugar are increased. Dr. Van Cauter limited eleven healthy men in their twenties to four hours of sleep for six straight nights, and she reports that it brought them to a nearly prediabetic state.

This unfortunate relationship between sleep—or lack of it— and hormones and metabolism cannot be underestimated by anyone who travels. Jet lag or no jet lag, the false signals will be there if you're not sleeping enough.

So how to fight it? Start with H_2O. Now, whenever I'm on the road and I feel hungry at a weird hour or at an interval that is too short between meals, I drink two 8-ounce bottles of water, and the hunger goes away. I have learned to recognize the false signals of hunger, and the water helps me counteract them.

In the end, it's not just about jet lag or how well you adjust. The bottom line is sleep deprivation and how that affects your ability to think clearly—and in particular, about food and how hungry you are, as opposed to how hungry you *feel*.

SLEEPING IN HOTELS

Thankfully, the hotel sleep and performance surveys are beginning to pay off for travelers: From pillow menus to bedtime music and even light therapy sessions, hotels are going the extra mile to ensure that guests get a good night's sleep.

BENJAMIN HOTEL

The Benjamin Hotel, a boutique hotel in New York City, is so serious about providing sweet dreams that guests can consult the hotel's very own sleep concierge, Eileen McGill. Eileen will get you snoring in no time, whether you need personalized pillow recommendations—there are ten types to choose from—or an in-room session of light therapy to help you fight jet lag. Additionally, guests can look forward to a night of slumber in the "Benjamin Bed," custom-designed in collaboration with Serta for the hotel. "It's the Goldilocks bed," says McGill, "not too hard, and not too soft; it's just right." But the best part of the Benjamin sleep experience? If you don't sleep like a baby, your night of tossing and turning Is on the house (www.thebenjamin.com)

CROWNE PLAZA

Rest assured, according to the folks at the Crowne Plaza, a good night's sleep is guaranteed—or your money back. Dr. Michael Breus, sleep disorder expert and cofounder of Sound Sleep, collaborated with the hotel to create its Sleep Advantage program, designed to help business and regular travelers sleep peacefully. According to Dr. Breus, travelers encounter two travel-related sleep conditions: the "first-night effect," stress from trying to sleep in an unfamiliar environment, and the "on-call effect," anxiety caused by worrying about waking up on time, or "will the alarm clock work?" syndrome.

Breus worked with the Crowne Plaza hotel chain to address these issues and develop the program. "Noise and light are two of the biggest factors when you are not going to get a good night's rest," says Breus. To help reduce sleep disruptions, the Crowne Plaza implemented "quiet zones" by instituting simple changes, such as altering housekeeping times to reduce noise. Other such fixes included adding nightlights in the bathrooms. "When you turn on the bathroom light in the middle of the night, the light is a signal in your mind to wake up," says Breus. The nightlight helps guests maintain their sleepy state.

Besides revamping their bedding and mattresses, the Crowne Plaza offers guests a sleep kit that includes earplugs, an eye mask, lavender spray, a sleep CD, a nightlight, and a drape clip to block out that annoying little sliver of light that always slips through the curtains. The hotel also offers guaranteed wake-up calls to ease travelers' nerves about missing that morning meeting. (www.ichotelsgroup.com)

FOUR POINTS
Four Points, the midrange Starwood brand, rolled out its new bedding line on Annual Napping Day in April. More than two hundred overworked New Yorkers walking down Fifth Avenue were offered a half-hour catnap in one of the newly designed Four Points beds. The Four Comfort Bed features a specially designed mattress, mattress pad, two feather/down pillows, and two oversized lounging pillows. (www.starwoodhotels.com)

HILTON
Hilton literally went to the mattress to ensure guests a thousand undisturbed winks. The Hilton

Suite Dreams bedding program custom-designed its mattress, adding coils to the middle of the mattress and 4 inches of height to reduce tossing and turning. Bedding has also been upgraded to new European-style, 250-thread-count linens, and the hotel has added extra pillows—double beds now get four pillows and kingsize beds get five.

Hilton has likewise custom-designed its own easy-to-set alarm clocks, putting them into all existing Hilton brands, including Hilton, Double-Tree, and Embassy Suites. (www.hilton.com)

HYATT

For business travelers too wired from a day of meetings to settle down for a nap or a good night's sleep, YogaAway, a Denver-based yoga company has teamed up with Hyatt to offer guests customized yoga programs attuned to travelers' ailments and complaints. Guests can access three different YogaAway programs on command from the comfort of their own hotel room. (www.yogaaway.com)

KIMPTON

At Kimpton's Hotel Burnham in Chicago, guests can choose a pillow from the hotel's pillow library, where the selection ranges from "Pillow-Positive," a pillow proven to reduce snoring, to the Sobagara (buckwheat hull) pillow, a natural and hypoallergenic pillow designed to increase circulation. However, if it's sweet dreams you are after, the hotel's herbalist has created a menu of herbal dream pillows, each of which was designed to promote a specific type of dream.

Kimpton's Hotel Monaco in Denver offers guests a complete bath menu. Guests can take a prebedtime soak in a Raw Lavender Tranquility Spa, a bath infused with lavender flowers, then rub down with lavender sugar scrub and body balm by the light of votive candles. Those looking for a more traditional bubble bath can try the SINsational, which comes with the girlie basics— a dirty martini, chocolate, gossip mags, and tons of bubbles. (www.kimptonhotels.com)

RADISSON

According to a survey conducted by Radisson Hotel & Resorts and Select Comfort, 55 percent of American adults would opt to bring their own bed on vacation if they could bring one comfort from home. To appease this majority, Radisson has teamed up with Select Comfort to offer the well-known Sleep Number bed to ensure that its guests are sleeping just the way they like to. The bed features adjustable air-chamber technology that allows guests to adjust each side of the bed to the firmness, or "sleep number," desired. (www.radisson.com)

RITZ-CARLTON

You can't be too careful about where you rest your head. At the Ritz-Carlton, Key Biscayne, picky sleepers can choose from twelve types of pillows, including down and foam-top, a hypoallergenic variety, and one that claims to help get rid of headaches.

But if you are just too wound up to fall asleep, the Ritz-Carlton, Naples, offers guests a signature rose-petal bath to soothe the stresses of the day. The bath is drawn for you and includes rose petals, rose bath salts, oil, a bath pillow, and a split of champagne that will surely help iron out the kinks of the day. (www.ritzcarlton.com)

"The quality and quantity of your sleep can make all the difference in how you function and feel each and every day," says Nancy Shark, spokesperson for the Better Sleep Council. "Even while traveling, you should take steps to ensure you get the best night's sleep possible."

Here are some simple rules from the Better Sleep Council to getting your zzzs on the road:

- If possible, adjust the room temperature. The ideal bedroom temperature is 60 to 65°F (16 to 18°C). A room that's too warm or too cool can disrupt sleep.

- If possible, make the room dark, quiet, and uncluttered. The rising sun can wake up the brain long before the alarm goes off and noise (such as a TV) can keep us from enjoying deep, restful sleep.

- Exercise regularly—yes, even while traveling. Make sure to complete your workout at least a few hours before bedtime. (The one thing that will help your performance: exercise. According to the Hilton study mentioned previously, travelers who exercised during their trip performed 61 percent better than nonexercisers when given a reaction and alertness test.)

- Avoid nicotine and caffeine close to bedtime and try to finish eating at least two to three hours before your regular bedtime.

SLEEPING ON PLANES

The airlines attempt to get you horizontal . . .

OVERSEAS CARRIERS

Air Canada
Some of Air Canada's long-haul international flights feature the completely flat Executive First bed, with ample storage space, lumbar support, a 21-inch seat, and a 63-inch pitch. Air Canada is introducing a lie-flat seat designed and manufactured by Contour Premium Aircraft Seating. The armchair and ottoman will recline into a truly lie-flat bed measuring 6 feet 3 inches (191 centimeters) long and up to 31 inches (79 centimeters) wide at the shoulders. (www.aircanada.com)

Air France
L'Espace Affaires (business Class) on Air France features seat beds that recline up to 131 degrees. The exterior shell of the bed shields passengers from aisle foot traffic. Air France has plans in the works to roll out a completely flat-lying seat bed. (www.airfrance.us)

Air New Zealand
Air New Zealand's new Business Premier service offers lie-flat beds that open up to 6 feet 7 inches, with a 22-inch-wide seat. A footrest doubles as a seat for visitors. (www.airnewzealand.com)

British Airways
BA was one of the first airlines to go absolutely horizontal. First-class and Club World (business-class) seats recline the full 180 degrees. The seat width itself is 20 inches, and the seat pitch — a.k.a. legroom — is a full 73 inches. (www.britishairways.com)

Lufthansa

Business travelers can enjoy a nearly flat Private-Bed. Seats recline to sleep mode at a 9-degree angle shy of horizontal. Additionally, the distance between seats has been increased from 30 centimeters (about a foot) up to 150 centimeters (almost 5 feet). (www.lufthansa.com)

Malaysia Airlines

Malaysia recently introduced flat seats on the B-747 and B-777 planes. As an added bonus, you can play around with the lumbar and seat positions. In-flight laptop adapters are available for use by first- and Golden Club–class passengers. Seats recline to 180 degrees, with a seat size of 19.8 inches and a pitch of 50 inches. (www.malaysiaairlinesusa.com)

Qantas

The new international business class cocoon-style Skybed is nearly flat, reclining to 172 degrees with a pitch of 60 inches. Additionally, the seat is 6 feet 6 inches in length. Other business-class amenities include noise-canceling headphones and a help-yourself snackbar. (www.qantas.com.au)

South African Airways

South African Airways has gone totally flat. Business passengers can enjoy a fully horizontal 180-degree recline with a seat width of 21 inches and a seat pitch of 73 inches. (www.flysaa.com)

Virgin Airlines

Richard Branson's airline introduced what it claims to be the "biggest totally flat seat" for its Upper-Class passengers. The seats recline 180 degrees into a totally private space, with a seat width of 22 inches and 33 inches wide at the shoulder area. Translation: Passengers get a full 2.5 more inches of width than the BA model that they won't let you forget about. On the A-340s there is even enough space for a baby to nap next to Mom. (www.virgin-atlantic.com)

MAJOR U.S. CARRIERS

American Airlines

AA is installing new lie-flat seats in the business-class cabin on all of the airline's Boeing 767-300 and Boeing 777 aircraft serving transatlantic routes. AA operates two different first-class cabin layouts aboard its B-777 flagship fleet: the sixteen-seat Flagship Suite and the larger, eighteen-seat configuration with lie-flat seats. (www.aa.com)

Continental

In Continental business class on the B-777, seats recline to 170 degrees, measuring 22 inches wide and extending 6½ feet. (www.continental.com)

Northwest Airlines

World Business Class offers cocoon-type beds that recline to 176 degrees. Additionally, seats are outfitted with lumbar support, a massager, and an adjustable headrest. (www.nwa.com)

United Airlines

Business-class seats recline to 150 degrees, with a seat width of 19 inches and a seat pitch of 55 inches. Seats also feature fully adjustable legs, back and seat rests, plus the Backcycler Motion System for lumbar support and back stimulation. (www.united.com)

CHAPTER 10

What I Learned: What Worked and What Didn't

Every man lies to himself.

—*Dostoyevsky*

In the interests of full disclosure and clarity, let's get this out of the way right now: I didn't always stick to the diet. With my intense schedule, both in the air and on the ground, I couldn't. And on a few days of intense travel and schedule disruptions . . . I *wouldn't*. And there were days I didn't get to the hotel gym, times I was late for my plane and didn't walk the entire length of an airport terminal, and yes, there was the occasional minibar that wasn't locked or removed and . . . I gave in and had that Snickers bar at two in the morning.

But on balance, I recovered from those lapses and stayed the course. I couldn't have lost the weight any other way. It was that combination of diet, exercise, and understanding about sleep that did the trick.

Most important, this was not just a project to see whether I could lose the weight, nor was it a short-term experiment, because if it was, it was/is doomed to failure. It is a nonnegotiable lifestyle change, a discipline that must be embraced now and into the future. To not do this would be to proceed at my own peril.

And along the way, I learned many things. Most ideas worked very well. Some worked occasionally. Very few approaches in this book were outright failures, and when they were, I've identified them. In all honesty, they were failures only because I chose not to use them. (This applies to certain exercises, pedometers, and food choices, outlined below).

DON'T MYTH THIS

First, so much of this program is about . . . movement. It's not about not eating or working out to the point of exhaustion. As Annette Lang told me, you don't have to break a sweat to improve. You just need to get moving any way you can. And that doesn't necessarily mean you need to work out an hour a day. Ten-minute bursts of exercise whenever you can are preferable to no exercise for three or four days. Recently, I was in San Francisco and found I had thirty minutes between two business meetings. Instead of hailing a cab, I walked fourteen blocks, and made the appointment on time. And that was at least half of my exercise for that day (the rest I did as routines in my hotel room).

Indeed, we have to overcompensate for the unhealthiness of travel. However, it's *not* a matter of no pain, no gain. That's a big, fat . . . lie. There really is a middle ground. In the end, it doesn't matter so much what you do as that you do *something*.

In fact, researchers at the Mayo Clinic figured out the key to low metabolism (simultaneously identifying a major factor in obesity). These researchers call it NEAT (for "nonexercise activity thermogenesis"), and it's a great way for you to gauge the number of calories you're actually burning outside of the gym routine. NEAT is the energy expended for everything we do that is not sleeping, eating, or regimented exercise. Remember, even trivial activities can increase metabolic rates substantially. We need to walk more, stand more, *move* more.

Here's the skinny: A sedentary life coupled with easy access to energy-dense food is the problem.

LOSING PROPOSITIONS

The other myth is that with more exercise, you burn more calories, and because of that, excess weight flies off effortlessly. Not true. There were a number of times during the course of this diet when, despite increased exercise activity, my weight plateaued. What I had to learn was that this is normal. On the road to my weight loss, I experienced at least six plateaus. These were not happy occasions for me. But after the second plateau, I learned to adjust to the bad mood that almost always immediately followed the plateau.

CHEAT ONCE A WEEK

This one was perhaps the simplest concept to embrace, with one important caveat. Not only is it OK to cheat once a week, but I quickly learned during one bad stretch that if I didn't cheat once a week, I ran a much higher likelihood of cheating all the time. Abstinence may be a virtue, but it makes absolutely no sense in the real world when it comes to eating and food. However, cheating once a week doesn't mean you get to cheat big—what it really means is that once a week, especially on the road, when you're offered a dessert, you can have it, in a small portion. That's the deal. Period.

EATING ON THE ROAD

Perhaps one of the most important things I've learned with the traveler's diet is discipline, with another important caveat. Rules are not sacred . . . but principles *are*. And the overriding principle with this diet, as with the process of travel itself, is common sense.

You already know that it's not easy to eat on the road. You often don't have control over where you'll be eating, when, or what will be served. But you *do* have control over how you eat and how much you consume at a given sitting.

What Can I Eat in the Parisian Café That's on My Diet?

Part of the pleasure of travel when you are in a different city or culture is to taste the local offerings. But *taste* is the key word. If you are in Paris and you want to try a fabulous dessert, take a cue from the locals. Those svelte Parisians will most likely sample the dessert, but they will not eat the whole thing. Follow Madelyn Fernstrom's advice: Indulge mildly.

Don't Skip Breakfast

Not everyone eats breakfast, and in many cultures, especially those in Europe, breakfast often consists of a piece of bread and a coffee. Standing up.

But researchers are uncovering more evidence that breakfast really is the most important meal of the day—especially when you're trying to lose weight. Making breakfast a routine can lower your chances of obesity by up to 50 percent. And eating a good breakfast has been associated with lower cholesterol levels and helping you eat foods that are lower in fat and cholesterol throughout the day.

This has become one of my biggest challenges. When I bolt out of bed in the morning, I hardly ever eat a great breakfast. And I probably never will. Instead, if I'm being good, I'll just eat an apple. But for the rest of you, follow the advice of the Mayo Clinic and eat a low-fat breakfast that emphasizes whole grains and fiber rather than skipping the morning meal. The Mayo Clinic recommends:

- Cereal: hot or cold, with a fiber content of 5 grams or more a serving, with skim milk.

- Fruit: Slice a banana on your cereal or grab an apple for the road.

An alternative, though it's not traditional, is to make a vegetable sandwich using whole-grain bread.

Don't Look at the Menu

When you eat out, simply order what you would like—grilled chicken, steamed vegetables, and rice, for example. And remember Anthony Scotto's advice: Be as specific and detailed as possible with your order, or that swordfish will come smothered in butter.

Perhaps a better idea is to eat everything you can with olive oil. Take the Mediterranean approach—not just for diet, but for pain relief! A study at the Monell Chemical Senses Center in Philadelphia discovered that olive oil contains a compound called oleocanthal that behaves like ibuprofen in the body, reducing inflammation and relieving pain. The research team further discovered that a daily intake of about 50 grams of olive oil contained the pain relief of 10 percent of a regular dose of Motrin.

Eat More Slowly

If you pay attention to what you're eating, you won't eat as much. It takes about twenty minutes for your stomach to realize it's full, so give it a chance to register.

Eat a Salad First

Eating a salad before your meal will help you eat less altogether, suggests a recent study from Pennsylvania State University. But be sure to ask for the dressing on the side. Then dip your fork into it before going for the leaves.

Watch Your Portions

Portions have gotten bigger. Some restaurants serve enough for two or three meals. If you question your willpower, ask them to wrap up half of the meal to go *before* you start. Or order from the children's or senior citizen's menus, to get smaller portions. A portion shouldn't be larger than your fist.

It's also a matter of simple equations using portion size and nutritional content. Michael Jacobson and Jayne Hurley, from the Center for Science in the Public Interest, did a terrific survey of restaurant and fast-food chain offerings in 2003. Their hit list, featuring calories, fat, and saturated fat, is worth noting.

Here are some highlights of their survey:

	Calories	Total Fat (grams)	Saturated Fat (grams)
Subway's "7 Subs with 6 grams of fat or less"	260	5	1
Blimpie Veggie Max Sub	400	7	1
McDonald's Fruit 'n Yogurt Parfait with granola	380	5	2
Turkey sandwich with lettuce, tomato, and mustard	370	6	2
Grilled or broiled chicken or seafood (average, without side dishes)	270	8	2
Szechuan shrimp or chicken with rice	930	19	2
Chicken, lamb, or pork souvlaki with rice	290	10	3
Chinese stir-fried spinach, broccoli, or mixed vegetables with rice	750	19	3
Pasta with red clam or marinara sauce	870	20	4
Fajitas (chicken, shrimp, or vegetable) with tortillas	840	24	5

And then there's the CSPI Restaurant Hall of Shame:

	Calories	Total Fat (grams)	Saturated Fat (grams)
Cheese fries with ranch dressing	3,010	217	91
Movie theater butter popcorn with "butter" topping (large)	1,640	126	73
Prime rib, untrimmed (16-ounce)	1,280	94	52
Fettuccine Alfredo	1,500	97	48
Stuffed potato skins with sour cream	1,260	95	48
Fudge brownie sundae	1,130	57	30
Beef and cheese nachos with sour cream and guacamole	1,360	89	28
Denny's Meat Lover's Skillet (ham, bacon, and sausage, over fried potatoes, with cheddar and two eggs)	1,150	93	26
The Cheesecake Factory (1 slice)	1,560	84	23
Pizzeria Uno Chicago Classic (1/2 pizza)	1,500	74	30

The charts that follow give you more information to help you make appropriate choices when you eat out.

Foods Lowest in Saturated Fat and Calories

Item	Calories	Saturated Fat (grams)
Panda Express Mixed Vegetables with Steamed Rice	300	0
Subway's "7 subs with 6 grams of fat or less" (6-inch)	260	1
Schlotzsky's Light and Flavorful Dijon Chicken Sandwich (small)	330	1
Broiled, blackened, or grilled seafood	270	1
Schlotzsky's Light & Flavorful Pesto Chicken Sandwich (small)	350	1
Blimpie Veggie Max Sub (6-inch)	400	1
Au Bon Pain Thai Chicken Sandwich	420	1
Hot or cold cereal with reduced-fat 2% milk	210	2
Wendy's Grilled Chicken Sandwich	300	2
Blimpie Turkey Sub (6-inch)	330	2
Schlotzky's Light & Flavorful Chicken Breast Sandwich (small)	360	2
Turkey sandwich with mustard	370	2
McDonald's Fruit 'n Yogurt Parfait with granola	380	2
Panda Express Chicken with Mushrooms with steamed rice	390	2
Blimpie Grilled Chicken Sub (6-inch)	400	2
Panda Express Chicken with String Beans with steamed rice	400	2
Au Bon Pain Honey Smoked Turkey Wrap	540	2

McDonald's McSalad Shakers with fat-free dressing	140	3
Taco Bell Chicken Soft Taco	190	3
Barbecue of grilled chicken breast	280	3
Taco Bell Chicken or Steak Gordita Nacho Cheese	290	3
KFC Tender Roast Sandwich	350	3
Blimpie Roast Beef Sub (6-inch)	390	3
Panda Express Beef & Broccoli with steamed rice	400	3
McDonald's Chicken McGrill Sandwich	450	3
Au Bon Pain Oriental Chicken Salad with light dressing	500	3
Crispy or soft chicken taco	220	4
Taco Bell Steak Soft Taco	280	4
Taco Bell Bean Burrito	370	4
Taco Bell Chicken or Steak Fiesta Burrito	380	4
Au Bon Pain Pesto Chicken Salad with light dressing	460	4
Roast beef sandwich with mustard	460	4

Foods Highest in Saturated Fat

Item	Saturated Fat (grams)
Cheese fries with ranch dressing	91
Fried whole onion with dipping sauce	57
Prime rib, untrimmed	*52*
Fettuccine Alfredo	48
Stuffed potato skins with sour cream	48
Porterhouse steak, untrimmed	40
The Cheesecake Factory Original Cheesecake	*31*

Fried mozzarella sticks	*28*
Burger King Double Whopper with Cheese	*27*
Cheese nachos	25
Taco Bell Mucho Grande Nachos	25
Cheese quesadillas with sour cream, pico de gallo, and guacamole	24
Au Bon Pain Sweet Cheese Danish	*23*
Onion rings	*23*
Burger King Double Whopper	*22*
Barbecue baby back ribs	*21*
Lasagna	21
Au Bon Pain Pecan Roll	*20*
Taco salad with sour cream and guacamole	20
Burger King Double Cheeseburger	19

Note: Aim for no more than 20 grams of saturated fat in a day. Less is better. Any single food with more than 4 grams of saturated fat should sound an alarm. Meat and full-fat dairy products explain the high levels of saturated fat in these foods. Saturated fat numbers in italics include artery-clogging trans fat.

Best Snacks

	Calories	Total Fat (grams)	Saturated Fat (grams)
Au Bon Pain fresh fruit cup	90	1	0
Häagen-Dazs Sorbet (1 scoop)	120	0	0
Auntie Anne's Original Pretzel, no butter	340	1	0
Starbucks Cappuccino with skim milk or			

Caffe Latte (grande—16-ounce)	140	1	1
Dunkin' Donuts Bagel with preserves	400	3	1
Au Bon Pain Low Fat Chocolate Cake or Low Fat Triple Berry Muffin	280	4	1
McDonald's Garden McSalad Shaker with Fat Free Herb Vinaigrette Dressing	140	6	3

Worst Snacks

	Calories	Total Fat (grams)	Saturated Fat (grams)
Sbarro Sausage and Pepperoni Stuffed Pizza (1 slice)	880	44	19
McDonald's shake (large)	1,010	29	19
Au Bon Pain Almond Croissant	630	42	18
Burger King french fries	600	30	16
Starbucks White Chocolate Mocha with whole milk (venti; 20-ounce)	600	25	15
Cinnabon	670	34	14
Dunkin' Donuts Bagel with cream cheese	540	22	14

Note: A snack is supposed to tide you over until lunch or dinner. Snacks such as a 670-calorie pastry or a 1,000-calorie shake have enough calories to be dinner.

Sandwiches

Remember that airport turkey wrap? As the CSPI's Jacobson and Hurley taught me in *Restaurant Confidential*, a little smear of mayonnaise instead of mustard doubles the total fat and boosts the calories by 100. And we all know there's more than just a little smear on that sandwich.

Seafood Strategy

- Pick a low-fat preparation method (baked, blackened, broiled, grilled, steamed).

- Beware of breading and batter (say goodbye to the coconut shrimp and the calamari).

- Hold the fries.

- Seek out healthy sides (skip the coleslaw and opt instead for a green salad).

- Say *hasta la vista* to biscuits.

Jacobson and Hurley have provided a comparison chart (page 321).

BACK AT THE HOTEL . . .

Here are a few last tips for making hotel visits part of the plan.

No Weigh

I've learned never to weigh myself on hotel scales. Not one of them has ever been accurate. You want to get depressed? Or overly confident? Stand on a hotel scale. Please, take my advice: Don't do it. Pick one scale—at your regular gym or at home—and depend only on that scale for your weight readings.

Entrées and platters	Calories	Total Fat	Saturated Fat	Cholesterol	Sodium
Appetizers:					
Steamed shrimp (3 ounces)	80	1	0	165	190
Steamed clams (3 ounces)	130	2	0	55	100
New England clam chowder (1.5 cups)	250	7	2	50	1,430
Entrées:					
Steamed lobster (3 ounces)	80	1	0	60	320
Steamed Alaska King Crab (3 ounces)	80	10	0	45	910
Broiled or grilled scallops (6 ounces)	150	3	1	65	990
Broiled low-fat fish (6 ounces)	210	5	1	125	360
Shrimp scampi (4 ounces)	150	5	2	230	550
Blackened catfish (6 ounces)	300	15	3	130	700
Broiled salmon (8 ounces)	420	21	4	155	340
Baked stuffed shrimp (8 ounces)	470	30	6	285	1,040
Fried fish (9 ounces)	520	24	8	145	840
Fried shrimp (7 ounces)	510	26	10	280	970
Fried clams (8 ounces)	830	47	19	65	1,660
Seafood casserole (12 ounces)	640	43	21	320	1,470

Lights Out

Then there's the lighting in that hotel room. When I check into a room, especially in the evening hours, or if I return to my hotel room after the housekeeper has done turn-down service, the very first thing I always do is open all the drapes and blinds. I want as much light in the room as possible. For me, it's not a food or exercise issue; I just know that when light comes into the room in the morning, it wakes me. Closed curtains—at least for me—mean I stand not just a very good chance of oversleeping, but a guaranteed one. I also find that keeping the curtains open and allowing natural light into the room helps my body adjust to local time.

But now, it seems there's an even better reason for allowing as much light into the room as possible. A study from the University of California at Irvine says that the darker the room, the higher the likelihood of overindulgence. And the reason: Brighter lighting forces you to be more aware of what you're eating . . .

A FEW FINAL WORDS ABOUT
WALKING . . . AND PEDOMETERS

You won't get an argument from me about walking. I'd choose walking through a city over walking on a treadmill any day. But I still don't do it enough.

Consider these facts: Research from the University of Colorado indicates that the average American man takes 6,733 steps a day (and 6,384 for women). But that's just the average. In Tennessee, for example, it's only 4,547 daily steps for men. West Virginia, Louisiana, and Mississippi were just as bad. But folks in Colorado, Montana, and Utah were, as they say, stepping out. And the average Amishman takes . . . 18,425 steps a day!

But those recommended thirty-minute walks may be overrated. University of Tennessee researchers (the same state where the men walk just over 4,500 steps a day) found that women who were told to take 10,000 steps a day walked more than those asked to take a half-hour walk. Why 10,000 steps? It appears to be a reasonable estimate of daily activity for healthy adults. And middle-aged women who took at least 10,000 steps a day have been found, on average, to be much more likely to fall into recommended ranges for body composition (total body weight and body fat percentage). The number of steps the women took were tracked using pedometers.

Over the course of twelve months, Annette Lang got me three different pedometers. I must admit I hated them. Either they didn't work or they gave false readings, or I would just forget to wear one.

Instead, I went back to the days when I was growing up in Manhattan, and I resumed walking city streets. I figured each city block was $\frac{1}{20}$ of a mile. Annette had measured my stride length at 2.3 feet. And I calculated my distances accordingly. Before long, I was walking a mile and a half every day—minimum. Now that might not seem like a lot, but it made a difference.

SO HOW DID I DO?

Between May 2005 and August 2005 I went from 284 pounds to 264 pounds.

In July, at my first workout, Annette measured me:

Chest	50.25 inches
Right arm	15.25 inches
Left arm	15 inches
Smallest part of waist	51 inches
Hips	48.75 inches

In November 2005, she did the second set of measurements:

Chest	48.5 inches
Right arm	15.125 inches

Left arm	14.875 inches
Smallest part of waist	45 inches
Hips	47.5 inches

I had lost 2½ inches from my chest. And a smile-inducing 6 inches from my waist!

By March I had lost another 2 inches from my chest and 2 inches off the waist. That was real progress.

My level of cardio exercise was definitely improving. Not just thirty minutes on the elliptical, but constant at Level 13, and burning around 400 to 450 calories per session. Treadmill was up to 3.8 miles per hour at 8- and 9-degree inclines.

And the Quickie? When I started, I was lifting around 6,000 pounds per workout. In October 2005 I was up to 9,835 pounds in twenty-four minutes. In January, my total had soared to 13,425! And Mark increased the lift/drop time to five seconds from four (that extra second is a killer—trust me).

By the middle of February, after my weight had once again plateaued, it started to drop again—and kept dropping. The key, as always, was consistent adherence to the workout plans, with both Annette and Mark.

By the time this book is published, I will have lost 44 pounds (from a high of 284 down to 240) and on the way to 224—for a loss of 60, exactly where I need to be. And all in just about a year.

I was doing eleven reps of 415 pounds on leg presses, eleven reps on leg curls at 75 pounds, and lat pulldowns . . . thirteen reps at 190 pounds! And the real killer—the abdominal crunches—had me doing nine reps (to failure) at 165 pounds.

A month later, the weights and reps were increased again—425 pounds and twelve reps on the leg presses, and the ab crunches— twelve reps (great improvement here) with an increase to 175 pounds.

WHAT DIDN'T WORK

I'm not a planner. To me *plan* is a bad four-letter word, something to *depart from*. And part of that stems directly from the travel experience. After all, so much of travel is about unexpected change and adjusting by going with plan B, C, or D. It's about keeping your options open.

So the odds were against me from the start. Still, I realized that I miss 100 percent of the shots I never take, so I gave it a try. And, slowly, surely, I was able to stick to the basic plan with this diet and exercise program. I cut out all the sweets. I ended my addiction to Diet Pepsi. I started as someone who was quite a nosher and tended not to eat real food—I usually opted for high calories and low nutrition—and I was the personification of the American epidemic: I was overweight and undernourished. Once I got with the program, I ended up eating better, eating less, and eating less often.

When I started the traveler's diet, I had high blood pressure and high cholesterol levels: My blood pressure was 145/95, and my cholesterol levels were over 200.

Nine months after starting the diet, my blood pressure was a remarkable 105/70, my total cholesterol was down to 165, and the LDL (bad cholesterol) levels were 65, down from nearly 95. My triglycerides had plummeted from 148 to 98.

Finally, an admission: I will never become a gym rat, but I was able to get into a semigroove with exercise. And in the end, coupled with a realistic and practical approach to eating, that's all I really needed to make it all work.

DIET ANOTHER DAY

Annette had to stay on me, probably more than she would have liked, to get me to finally adopt a rhythm of exercise and diet that made sense.

To her credit, she never asked me to be a fitness zealot. There are no magic exercises. I just needed to get my body moving more, and Annette accomplished that in a variety of ways by giving me a flexible program that incorporated different options. Traveling, by definition, encompasses a sense of movement and being mobile and active—so I had that going for me.

At the same time, she forced me to be honest with myself. Did I like and respect myself enough to make some changes? It was—and remains—a mind-set. After all, as Yogi Berra once said, "Half this game is 90 percent mental."

CHAPTER 11

Resources

These are just a few of the great organizations and groups that helped me with the research for this book and pointed me in the right direction. Most of the websites are user-friendly. I used them often, and in combination, to help keep me on the traveler's diet. I hope they help you as well.

ORGANIZATIONS

American Council on Exercise (ACE)
4851 Paramount Drive
San Diego, CA 92123
858-279-8227 or 800-825-3636
www.acefitness.org

As the world's largest nonprofit fitness certifying organization, the American Council on Exercise (ACE) promotes the benefits of physical activity and sets education standards for fitness professionals. If you're looking for an ACE-certified personal trainer or a fitness instructor in your area, visit this website and search by zip code. The site also offers fitness tips and exercise Q&As.

American Dietetic Association (ADA)
120 South Riverside Plaza, Suite 2000
Chicago, IL 60606-6995
800-877-1600
www.eatright.org

The ADA provides nutrition information, resources, and access to registered dieticians. Check out the ADA homepage to find contact information for registered dieticians in your area, or call for a referral. The ADA has also compiled nutritional fact sheets and tips on their website.

American Heart Association (AHA)
National Center
7272 Greenville Avenue
Dallas, TX 75231
800-AHA-USA-1 or 800-242-8721
www.americanheart.org

The AHA website is full of nutritional advice, recipes, and information about diet and exercise.

Centers for Disease Control and Prevention (CDC)
1600 Clifton Road
Atlanta, GA 30333
800-311-3435
www.cdc.gov

The CDC provides travelers with health warnings and advice for travel around the world. Log on to their website for up-to-date country-specific info, from virus outbreaks to recommended shots and medical precautions for travelers.

Center for Science in the Public Interest (CSPI)
875 Connecticut Avenue NW, Suite 300
Washington, DC 20009
202-332-9110
www.cspinet.org

This nonprofit organization provides nutritional information about the food available in restaurants and fast-food restaurants. The center's book, *Restaurant Confidential*, by Michael F. Jacobson, PhD, and Jayne Hurley, RD, is a wake-up call about the number of calories your restaurant meals really contain. CSPI's *Eating Smart Restaurant Guide* is a portable way to keep track of what you're eating, listing the calories, fat, and transfat numbers for more than 250 restaurant and fast-food chains.

National Sleep Foundation
1522 K Street NW, Suite 500
Washington, DC
202-347-3471
www.sleepfoundation.org

The National Sleep Foundation is a nonprofit organization whose mission is to promote public understanding of sleep disorders and to support sleep-related education, research, and advocacy to improve public health and safety. Their website is a forum for all things sleep related, including tips for treating jet lag and insomnia.

FOOD/NUTRITION

http://hin.nhlbi.nih.gov/menuplanner/menu.cgi

If you have the patience to enter each component of a meal, the National Heart, Lung, and Blood Institute's Menu Planner is for you. It allows you to enter the number of servings you want and then tallies up your total calories for your meal. It also allows you to plan out your day ahead of time so you'll stay within your calorie limit.

www.vegdining.com

At this website you'll find a guide to more than a thousand vegetarian restaurants around the world.

www.happycow.net

Happy Cow allows you to browse vegetarian and vegetarian-friendly restaurants around the world, as well as health food stores so you can buy healthy snacks for the road.

www.healthy-dining.com

This site is devoted to providing nutrition information for restaurant meals. It is useful in helping you decide where to eat when you have to eat out. Although it focuses mainly on restaurants in California, there is some information on various chain restaurants as well.

www.gayot.com

This website offers a list of heart-healthy restaurants (click on "Health" and then "Healthy Dining").

www.nutrition.gov

Nutrition 101 from the federal government. From the bottom of the food pyramid on up, this site provides more than a thousand links to current and reliable nutrition information, including food safety and science-based dietary guidelines. Additionally, specialized nutrition information is provided about the needs of infants, children, teens, adult women and men, and seniors.

www.heartriskevaluations.com/test.htm

How healthy are you? If you know your cholesterol level, blood pressure, and fasting blood sugar, this site will help you determine your risk for a heart attack. The site will show how you compare to the average American. Plus, you'll get tips on how to reduce your risk.

www.healthfinder.gov

This site provides detailed information on basic health and wellness. Its Health Library features dictionaries, encyclopedias, and journals relating to medical issues. Its search page helps connect people with organizations that address their specific concerns.

www.helpguide.org

This website offers expert information on wellness issues. Follow the links to Healthy Eating or Staying Sharp & Fit and learn about topics such as healthy fast-food choices and general guidelines for eating out.

www.pdrhealth.com

This is a general health/wellness website that offers eating advice and secrets to healthy restaurant dining, including questions to ask your waitstaff and ways to make certain menus and meals work better for your diet.

DIET/CALORIE COUNTERS

www.nal.usda.gov/fnic/foodcomp/search

Want to know what's in your food? The USDA Nutrient Database lets you search thousands of common foods and beverages for their nutritional makeup. It also includes fast-food offerings such as McDonald's and Burger King french fries.

www.cdc.gov/nccdphp/dnpa/5aday/month/index.htm

To inspire you to eat your fruits and vegetables, the CDC highlights one fruit and one vegetable each month. They also give you tips on how to prepare and store them.

www.thedietchannel.com/Diet-Menus.htm

This site offers detailed information on every type of diet, from Atkins to the Peanut Butter Diet. It includes dozens of nutrition calculators and diet articles. Click on a diet name and you can read an overview of the diet, including its success rate. The site also features a listing of daily menus based on food type, with a precalculated calorie content for dieters to follow on a day-to-day basis.

www.dietfacts.com

This site provides nutritional information for hundreds of restaurants. Most of the places listed are chain restaurants that travelers may encounter when they are out of town.

www.nhlbisupport.com/bmi

This site helps you calculate your body mass.

HEALTH ON THE ROAD

www.travelean.com

This website is designed to help with "weight management for corporate travelers." It offers tools that allow travelers to calculate their BMI, their caloric intake, and their activity levels as a guideline for keeping themselves fit on the road. The site also provides daily logs where you can record the foods you've eaten, the calories consumed, and the exercise completed.

www.healthytravelnetwork.com

This site features up-to-date travel fitness news and lists a variety of products that are useful for en-route exercise routines. The site also includes tips for flying fit, staying fit, and dining fit. Each tip is given with detailed warnings and lists of what to eat, what to avoid, and how to work out while traveling. The site also offers tools such as the Fitness Hotel Finder, along with a Travel Fitness blog. Articles on the latest healthy travel topics are also provided in the form of a monthly newsletter.

www.travelfitness.com

This site presents a list of travel tips, along with quizzes to identify your level of fitness as a traveler, and specific packing lists for varying diet, fitness, and health needs. The site also provides a list of links to diet and travel resources and books and illustrates several exercises recommended for before and after travel. The tips are based on the contents of the book *Travel Fitness: Feel Better, Perform Better on the Road,* by Rebecca Johnson and Bill Tulin.

EXERCISE

www.crossfit.com

Police academies and military special ops units are just a few of the fitness fanatics that use CrossFit's strength and conditioning program. Civilians trying to get fit can go to the site's workout of the day, such as the "Murph": 1-mile run, 100 pull-ups, 200 push-ups, 300 squats, and another 1-mile run.

www.airportgyms.com

Looking for a gym close to an airport? Start at this site, but don't necessarily depend on it. Just beware that many of the independent gyms the site lists are no longer in business, so be sure to call ahead and confirm that the gym is still there.

www.aapsm.org

Looking for the perfect athletic shoe to take with you? The American Academy of Podiatric Sports Medicine updates its list of favorite running shoes every three months or so. It also gives you tips on fitting the right shoe to your foot.

www.ballyfitness.com

This site maps out Bally Total Fitness Club locations in the United States and Canada.

www.24hourfitness.com

To find locations in the United States, Hong Kong, Malaysia, Singapore, and Taiwan, use the Find a Club feature.

www.goldsgym.com

Find six hundred gyms in twenty-seven countries with their Find a Gym feature.

www.ymca.net

Access this site to find thousands of YMCA locations in the United States and abroad.

www.runnersworld.com

This is the site for all things running, from trails and races around the country, to how to measure your pace. You can even get tips for running-friendly hotels.

www.swimmersguide.com

This most comprehensive guide lists around sixteen thousand publicly accessible, full-size, year-round swimming pools in 155 countries.

www.hotelfitnessclub.com

This site will help you search cities and airports for hotels with fitness clubs.

www.healthclubs.com

A service of the International Health, Racquet and Sportsclub Association (IHRSA) Passport Program, this site allows you to look up health clubs in cities across the country and abroad. The site also provides information on amenities and guest passes. IHRSA established the Passport Program to give members of participating IHRSA clubs guest privileges in over three thousand clubs worldwide when traveling. Most clubs will charge a guest fee per visit. The site also includes gyms that aren't members of the program.

www.justmove.org

Sponsored by the American Heart Association, this site supports you as you exercise with a digital diary, weekly updates, and an opportunity to hear from other exercise devotees.

www.gorp.com

If you are the adventurous type, this site has tools to help outdoor travelers plan active vacations.

http://win.niddk.nih.gov/publications/physical.htm

The Weight-Control Information Network, an information service of the National Institute of Diabetes and Digestive and Kidney Diseases (NIDDK), provides information on weight control, obesity, physical activity, and related nutritional issues.

www.shapeup.org

Shape Up America! is a not-for-profit organization committed to raising awareness of obesity as a health issue. Shape Up America! aims to provide evidence-based information and guidance on weight management to the public, health care professionals, educators, policymakers, and the media. Shape Up America! has recently expanded its mission to include reducing the incidence and prevalence of childhood obesity in America.

www.velonews.com

This site offers a comprehensive cycling guide.

www.fitnessonline.com

This site functions as a general resource for all areas of fitness facts. It has links to all kinds of fitness calculators including those for BMI, weight loss potential, ideal weight, calories, and sleep. The site offers tips, workout routines, and advice on how to exercise and eat right.

ALTERNATIVE MODES OF TRAVEL

> It is by riding a bicycle that you learn the contours of a country best, since you have to sweat up the hills and coast down them. Thus you remember them as they actually are, while in a motor car only a high hill impresses you, and you have no such accurate remembrance of country you have driven through as you gain by riding a bicycle.
> —*Ernest Hemingway*

The easiest way to incorporate exercise into your trip is to make it part of your trip. Instead of hailing a cab to explore the city you're visiting, why not hop on a couple of wheels. Many hotels across the country are now offering their guests free wheels—bike tires, that is. Besides being an affordable mode of transportation, biking around town is a great way to get some extra exercise and a surefire way to get to know the city you are visiting.

Here is just a sample of places you can rent or borrow a bicycle.

Austin

Four Seasons Austin
Ride the path around Town Lake. The hotel's health club rents bicycles to guests at a rate of $10 an hour including helmets, bike locks, and a trail map. (512-478-4500, www.fourseasons.com/austin)

Boston

Royal Sonesta Hotel
Bike rental is free the first two hours at the Royal Sonesta Hotel and only $5 for each additional hour. Bikes are on loan every summer from June until Labor Day. After Labor Day, the bikes go into hibernation until the summer sun is shining again. (617-806-4200, www.sonesta.com/boston)

Chicago

Drake Hotel
Take a spin along the Lakefront. The Drake Hotel is located a hop, skip, and jump from the Lake Michigan shoreline, where cyclists can ride on a bike path for 26 miles north. Bike rentals are just $20 for three hours. Additionally, the concierge will provide a map and get you the inside scoop on the best beach spots for a picnic. (312-787-2200, www.thedrakehotel.com)

Denver

Omni Interlocken Resort
Bike around the Interlocken trails for free. The Omni Spa loans out bikes, helmets, and trail maps to guests free of charge. You don't need to be a mountain-biking maven to negotiate the trails. Every trail is marked for level of difficulty, from novice to mountain-biking maniac. (303-438-6600, www.omnihotels.com)

Kauai

Hyatt Regency Kauai Resort and Spa

Take in the garden island by bike. The folks at the Hyatt Tennis Pro Shop will outfit you with bikes, helmets, locks, and plenty of advice on where to go. Many bikers head out to Spouting Horn, a natural wonder that spouts water 50 feet into the air, or to one of the secluded beaches around the island. Mountain bike rentals run $25 for two hours, or $35 all day. (808-742-1234, http://kauai.hyatt.com)

Los Angeles

Ritz-Carlton, Marina Del Rey

Bike alongside the serene Pacific, feet from the beach. The hotel is located minutes from a bike trail, which will take you from Venice Beach all the way to Malibu. Take in the local surf culture, musclemen, and maybe even a volleyball game or two. The cost is $15 per hour, $40 per half day, and $55 for an entire day. The hotel provides maps, and the staff will give you the skinny on the best places to dismount and take in some of the sights. (310-823-1700, www.ritzcarlton.com/hotels/marina_del_rey)

Venice Beach Suites & Hotel

This hotel, located right on the Ocean Front Walk in Venice Beach, offers guests a special bike rental package. The package includes a 10 percent discount on all forms of wheels—bikes, boards, or blades—a bike pack that includes soda or water, a power bar, and fresh fruit, plus late checkout and complimentary luggage storage.

Jay's Rentals (310-392-7306) rents out bikes to guests at discounted prices—just $15 for an all-day beach cruiser or BMX bike. (888-877-7602, www.venicebeachsuites.com)

San Diego

Holiday Inn on the Bay

Cycling enthusiasts, you have come to the right place. The Holiday Inn on the Bay boasts a bike shop on the hotel premises that rents out beach cruisers for $10 an hour or mountain bikes for $12. Additionally, a half-day rental is just $24. Cruise along the boardwalk or take your bikes on the ferry to Coronado Island. For just a $5.50 fare, you are free to explore the island. All rentals include bike helmets and locks. (619-232-3861, http://hisandiego-onthebay.felcor.com)

Washington, D.C.

Four Seasons

Bike along the Potomac River, and take a serene break from the hectic capital city. With just a day or two of notice, the Four Seasons will arrange for bikes that fit your measurements to be brought to the hotel. Bikes run anywhere from $38 to $48, depending on type. Maps and tips on where to go are also provided. Both come free of charge. (202-342-0444, www.fourseasons.com/washington)

Biking lets you get up close and personal with the people, culture, and landscape of your vacation destination. Just ask John Gill, avid cyclist, explorer, and president of Escape Travel. "You will see things that you wouldn't necessarily see on your own—back roads and byways, walks through old growth redwood forests," says Gill. Escape Travel was born out of Gill's love of outdoor travel. Gill would take friends and family on personalized hiking and biking tours of Northern California.

"I thought, if I could do this with friends and family, why not with others?" Gill explains. Escape Travel now operates cycling and multisport adventures throughout Northern California, including a wine-tasting tour of Sonoma County. Guests cycle anywhere from 17 to 26 miles each day, stopping along the way at cafés, old-growth forests, and, of course, wineries.

But you don't have to be an iron man to enjoy the journey, Gill is quick to reassure. "We are not concerned about time, distance, or speed—this is a vacation after all," he says. Two guides accompany the cyclists, with a van trailing behind for anyone too tired or tipsy to complete the daily ride. "Vacation with some exercise" is Escape's slogan. "Everyone can challenge themselves as little or much as they want." And the best part about working out all day is that you can go ahead and order that big steak for dinner—you've earned it.

From the vineyards of Northern California to the rice paddies of China, bike tours are being offered virtually everywhere in the world. Here are some great exercise journeys that will get you behind the handlebars.

Escape SF Tours

Bike through Sonoma wine country on this three-day, multi-sport trip with Escape SF Tours. Stop for some wine tasting as you wind through the vineyards around Lake Sonoma, and even cross the Golden Gate Bridge. Escape SF also offers a four-day multisport package that includes kayaking and hiking in the itinerary. (www.escapesftours.com)

Huck Finn Adventure Travel

It's hard not to hum *The Sound of Music* show tunes as you cycle through the Slovenian Alps. On Huck Finn Adventure's eight-day tour, cyclists will get to ride to Vrsic Pass for afternoon tea and a snack in the hut over 1,600 meters above sea level, cycle to Bohinj Lake, follow the green Sava Bohinjka River to Bled Lake, picnic and rest by the river and Pericnik waterfall, and much more. (http://ecotourism.gordonsguide .com/huckfinn)

Bike China Adventures

You can join the millions of Chinese who use bikes as their main form of transport on a seventeen-day, sixteen-night bicycle tour through China. Start off in Beijing and bike through the country, visiting Tiananmen Square, the Great Wall, the Forbidden City, the Terracotta Warriors, and the pandas at the Wolong Nature Reserve. Then cycle 31 kilometers down to Rilongguan at the base of the Four Sisters Mountains, and finally wind up in Shanghai. The tour includes a guide, hotel accommodations, meals, a bicycle, and travel insurance for the duration of the tour. (www.bikechina.com)

Skyline Overseas Treks and Cycle Rides

For a more exotic adventure, Skyline Overseas offers bike trips around locations such as Peru, the Sahara, London, and Vietnam. Local guides (as well as bike mechanics) will escort you through the French countryside or the wilderness of Iceland. But even better news is that you may be able to bike for charity. Travelers can participate for free by raising sponsorship money for various charities. Easy instructions on how to raise money are provided by Skyline. (www.skylineoverseas.co.uk)

Maui Downhill

You can almost feel the rush of the lava as you experience the free spirit of Hawaii, zooming downhill on Haleakala Volcano. Maui Downhill offers visitors a variety of biking tours of the island's volcano sights and tropics, including the ever-popular Haleakala trek, where you coast 38 miles downhill. Sunset tours are also available for those who have packed their day with activities. (www.mauidownhill.com)

Escape Adventures

Mountain bike the old Arizona trail through the Grand Canyon on Escape Adventures' four-day mountain-biking excursion around the rim of the Grand Canyon. Ride through Ponderosa forests and Aspen glens while enjoying the views of the canyon that you simply won't see from the car window. (www.escape adventures.com/tours/mountain_bike_tours)

Here are some other ideas for trips built around getting into better shape.

Southern Sea Ventures Sea Kayak Holidays

Southern Sea Ventures offers kayaking vacations that can be taken in areas that range from the Arctic to Australia. Travelers are escorted by a kayaking guide in groups of eight to ten throughout various tropical or polar regions. Trips are taken aboard the mothership Polar Pioneer, which acts as a base camp and holds a fleet of kayaks. Camping is also a part of the excursion. Trips generally range from one to two weeks at a cost of about $3,000 to $5,000, not including airfare. (+61 2 8901 3287, www.southernseaventures.com)

Fatpacking

This organization offers one- to two-week weight-loss backpacking trips all over the United States. Backpackers may choose to trek the California coastline or the canyons of Arizona. Participants are usually between 15 and 50 pounds overweight and range from age twenty-one to sixty. Although hikers are encouraged to eat what they want, they often lose between 5 and 15 pounds, carrying heavy loads as they travel. Trips are led by "nonintimidating" guides and cost between $750 and $1,000. (781-773-1115, www.fatpacking.com)

Spafari

Calling itself a "traveling adventure spa," Spafari is available in Africa, Indonesia, Arizona, Italy, Colorado, England, New Zealand, California, and many more locations. The experience includes yoga, day hikes, cultural expeditions, and massages, and combines the luxury of the spa with fitness challenges and cultural excursions. Spafari also offers customized vacations and special senior packages. Participants travel in small groups and stay at intimate locations that include haciendas, lodges, ranches, and villas, which are all run by the Spafari staff. Trips feature "zone"-style gourmet health cuisine, and they last one to two weeks, for a cost of about $3,000 to $5,000. (970-927-2882, www.globalfitnessadventure.com)

The World Outdoors

The World Outdoors offers private trips, multisport adventures, and hiking tours all over the world. You can hike, bike, kayak, and snorkel for six days all around the Hawaiian islands, canoe in Southern France, or ride in a hot-air balloon over Tuscany. Guides are expert instructors, so the skill level of participants can range from beginner to expert. Trips cater to families as well as elderly travelers, in groups of about ten people with a seven-to-one ratio of guests to guides. All meals, equipment, and lodging are provided and included in the price of each adventure. Trips last from one to two weeks and cost $1,000 to $3,000. (800-488-8483, www.theworldoutdoors.com)

Adventuresports.com

This claims to be the "World's #1 Active Travel Company." Both camping and hotel-centered trips are available for people of all ages. Multisport, hiking, and biking adventures are offered through Asia, Europe, Africa, and the United States. They are designed to accommodate people with varying levels of physical fitness. To plan your trip, you must call and consult a fitness travel agent, who will help you find the perfect vacation for your particular needs. Each trip lasts about a week and costs between $2,000 and $5,000. (510-527-1555, www.adventuresports.com)

MountainFit
This is a San Francisco–based company that offers hiking vacations in Montana, Utah, and Hawaii. MountainFit is a traveling spa designed to physically challenge travelers. (www.mountain fit.com)

Adventure Hyatt
At the Hyatt Beaver Creek, fitness is an outdoor affair—a Colorado hiking adventure with a cushy base camp. Included in Hike Week packages are four nights' lodging; reflexology or stone massage; use of hiking poles, shoes, and inclement-weather gear, and professional hiking guides; and transportation to trailheads. Single-occupancy packages are $1,625; double-occupancy is $1,285 per person. (http://beavercreek.hyatt.com)

Remarkable Adventures New Zealand
This company offers multiactivity adventure tours for people of moderate fitness that include glacier hiking, jet boating, whitewater rafting, cave rafting, hiking, and sailing. Tours last from one to two weeks and are offered throughout the year, for a cost between $1,500 and $4,000. (www.remarkableadventuresnz.co.nz)

Sheri Griffith Expeditions
On a rafting excursion in Colorado or Utah, you'll spend three to six days kayaking or rafting on the river of your choice, and nights camping on its riverbank. Trips include all food, beverages, and equipment. Tours maintain a one-to-six ratio of guides to participants. Travelers can participate in a variety of multisport activities, for prices ranging from $300 to $1,000. (www.griffithexp.com)

Exposure Alaska
Custom-plan an active one-week Alaskan adventure. Guides lead groups of no more than six on a tour that includes sea kayaking, glacier tours, and ice climbing. No experience is required of

participants, and the tour promises "less travel time in a van." All meals and equipment are included. (www.exposurealaska.net)

But what if you don't want to make your whole trip an exercise experience, but you'd like to incorporate some exercise into the package? Here are some ways to do this, making it fun at the same time.

Arizona

Arizona Climbing and Adventure School
Take a one-day beginner rock-climbing course for $125 per person. Classes are offered on Thursdays and Saturdays in groups of three or four. (www.climbingschool.com)

Salt River Canyon Whitewater Trips
This company offers one-day, overnight, and three-day whitewater rafting trips, from two and a half hours out of Phoenix in a unique location where sights include wild desert flowers and Indian ruins. The cost of an overnight trip is $325 per adult. (800-462-7238, www.inaraft.com/salt-river-arizona-2day.htm)

Atlanta

High Country Rock Climbing
One- or two-day rock-climbing excursions and lessons are available through High Country in the Atlanta area. Prices for lessons are $245 a day for one person and $295 for two people. Backpacking trips are $100 for one day and $150 for two days. (404-814-0999, www.highcountryoutfitters.com)

Boston

Appalachian Mountain Club—Boston Division
The Boston Division of the AMC offers year-round weekend hiking trips in the Boston area. (http://world.std.com/~bostonhb/activities.html)

Boston Bike Tours

This company takes you on fun sightseeing tours through Boston and Cambridge. Tours are slow-paced, mostly following bike paths through Boston's pretty parks. (617-308-5902, www .bostonbiketours.com)

Essex River Basin Adventures

ERBA offers kayaking tours to paddlers of all levels. The tours last from two to five hours at a cost of $25 to $75. There is also a four-day kayak training program, called Soup to Nuts Basic Kayak Training. During this session participants learn strokes and safety skills, for $250 per person. (www.erba.com)

Chicago

Bike Chicago

Bike Chicago provides day and night bike tours of the Windy City. Customers can choose a guided or self-guided tour. Guided tours take you through Chicago's main parks, stopping at fountains, gardens, and even the zoo. Bikes rent for as low as $9.99 a day. (312-595-9600)

Bobby's Chicago Bike Hike

Take a day or night bike tour of Chicago for $30. (www.bobbys bikehike.com)

Colorado

Colorado Adventures

Colorado Adventures offers one-, two-, and three-day whitewater rafting trips in several locations throughout Colorado. Price varies based on length of trip, but can range from about $300 to $500. (www.inaraft.com/colorado-adventure-trips.htm)

Florida

Crystal Seas Kayaking Tours
Crystal Seas offers two to seven days of kayaking and camping in Florida's Everglades as well as customized tours throughout the Florida Keys. For two days and one night, the cost is $319 per person. (877-SEAS-877, www.crystalseas.com/florida/multi-day.html)

Florida Surf Lessons
Learn how to surf safely, and get in shape at the same time (www.floridasurflessons.com)

Los Angeles

Daniel's Bike Rentals
Daniel's offers bike rentals seven days a week from Marina Del Rey. Mountain bikes are available for bike trips to the Santa Monica Mountains, and regular bikes are available for beach trails and other jaunts. Rentals run $20 to $30. (310-980-4045)

Learn to Surf LA
Learn to surf anywhere from Santa Monica to Malibu. Take three one-on-one lessons for $300. The school guarantees you will be up and surfing on your first lesson! It also offers an on-location masseuse with each lesson. (310-663-2479, http://learntosurfla.com)

Maui

Hike Hawaii
Take a full- or half-day hiking tour of Maui's waterfalls, mountains, and rain forests. Hike Hawaii also offers snorkeling and kayaking trips at a price that ranges from $65 to $150. (866-324-MAUI, www.hikemaui.com)

Maui Kiteboarding
For something truly alternative, try kiteboarding lessons in Maui. Lessons can last from three to nine hours at a cost of $200 to $500 per session. (http://mauikiteboardinglessons.com)

New York

Bear Cub Adventure Tours

Near Lake Placid, you can take weekend tours for kayaking, skiing, canoeing, and more. They even offer Winter and Summer Weekend Survival Adventures, on which travelers learn how to survive in the wilderness. Price varies between $700 and $1,000 for a couple. (518-523-4339, http://mountain-air.com/canoeing/ratetrips)

Weekend Warrior Tours

If you're a weekend warrior, this company offers full weekends of hiking, biking, kayaking, and general fitness training are offered in the Hamptons area. (631-267-2274, www.weekendwarriortours.com)

Acknowledgments

When it came to researching, reporting, and writing this book, there were no slim pickings. Stephen Perrine at *Best Life* was instrumental in first supporting the idea and then delivering the people to make it happen: Nutritionist Heidi Skolnik got me started eating right, and trainer Annette Lang, a great teacher and an unflinching cheerleader, never quit on me, even when I sometimes lapsed into bad exercise patterns.

Laura Hubber, who is also editor of my online travel newsletter for NBC, worked tirelessly to track down information and experts, and her attention to detail and follow-through were amazing. She performed the Herculean task of assembling all the material, then making sure it wasn't just factual but that it actually made sense. I'm convinced she lost weight just working on this book! She's now off on a well-deserved sabbatical of world travel (and of course, healthy eating).

Special thanks to Bruce Tracy, my editor, who bravely hangs in there with me as deadlines approach, pass, and, well . . . let's just say, he's quite brave. My agent, Amy Rennert, was always there to guide me through the maze. And thanks to Ginny Carroll, who was the real navigator in the home stretch, with copy-editing and structure, as she has been with many of my other books. Ginny is an indispensable gem.

Thanks also to Betsy Alexander at the *Today* show, who continues to shine as a beacon of good (and common) sense, without whose support this book never would have happened.

Then there's my research staff, Nina Porzucky, Matt Calcara, and Sarika Chawla, who stayed up late most nights tracking down airport and airline information, verifying quotes and data from around the world, and then double-checking accuracy. That wasn't always easy, since very little exercise and menu information was readily available—either at airports or from airlines—and wading through hotel menus without expert guidance proved useless.

Special thanks goes to Harvey Hopson, Food and Beverage Manager at Cleveland Hopkins Airport, who went beyond the call of duty to track down every available kernel of nutritional information about his vendors.

Thanks also to:

Felicia Browder, Media Relations Manager, Atlanta Hartsfield-Jackson Airport

Phil Orandella and the Massport Public Affairs Department

Wendy Abrams, Assistant Commissioner, Media Relations, City of Chicago

Ted Bushelman, Director of Communications, Cincinnati/Northern Kentucky International Airport

Dallas–Fort Worth Airport Public Affairs Department

Chuck Cannon, Manager of Public Affairs, Denver International Airport

Public Affairs Department, Detroit International Airport

Gallatin Field Airport Authority and Overland Express Restaurant, Bozeman, Montana

Grand Rapids Airport Public Affairs Department

Roger Smith, Public Affairs, Houston-Bush Intercontinental Airport

Judi O'Donnell, Senior Properties Specialist, Kansas City International Airport

Elaine Sanchez and Debbie Millett, Public Affairs, McCarran Airport, Las Vegas

Gaby Pacheco and the LAX Public Affairs Office, Los Angeles World Airports

General Mitchell Airport Management, Milwaukee

Manchester Airport Management, New Hampshire

Miami International Airport Public Affairs Department

Patrick Hogan, Spokesman, Metropolitan Airports Commission, Minneapolis

Monterey Airport and the Golden Tee Restaurant

Margherite LaMorte, Marketplace Development, LaGuardia Airport

Cara Marino, the Marino Organization, for JFK Airport

New York Port Authority Public Affairs Department

Public Affairs Department, Orlando International Airport

Julie Rodriguez, Public Affairs, Phoenix Sky Harbor

Richmond Airport Public Affairs

Barbara Gann, Director of Public Affairs, Salt Lake City

Savannah Airport Commission

Springfield-Branson Airport Management

Mike McCarron, Director of Community Affairs, SFO

Courtney Prebech, Spokeswoman, Washington, D.C., Airport Authority

Yeager Airport Management, Charleston, West Virginia

Special thanks goes out to the many people at the following international airports, who overcame time zones, language barriers, and cultural differences to deliver me much-needed inside information.

First, thanks to the Airports Council International's Manager of Communications, Nancy Gautier, for helping track down many of the following very helpful people around the world who could give up-to-the-minute answers.

Marianne de Bie, Press Office, Schiphol Group, Amsterdam

Haldane Dodd, Public Affairs, Auckland International Airport

Natalie Figueroa, Generencia de Comunicaciones, Aeropuertos Argentina

Communications Department, Airports Company South Africa

Shamma Majid Lootah, Manager, Press Relations and Communications, Department of Civil Aviation, Dubai

Ciara Carroll, External Communications, Dublin Airport

Chris Lam, Communications, Hong Kong Airport

Heathrow Airport Media Centre

Goksu Ozavcy, Press Relations Specialist, Istanbul

Adelina Rwelamira, Communications Department, Johannesburg Airport

Shuhainie Shamsudin, Director of Public Relations, Kuala Lumpur

Stephanie LePage, Media Relations, Montreal

Sergey Tanashchuk, Press Secretary, Eastline Group, Moscow

Erica Gingerich, International Media Relations, Munich

Mathieu Monnet, Responsable Presse, Aeroports de Paris

Olafur Ragnars, Chief of Department, Civil Aviation Administration, Reykjavik

Mafalda Bruno, Press Office, ADR, Rome

Suchin Pay, Communications, Seoul Airport

Satwinder Kaur, Public and International Relations Manager, Changi Airport, Singapore

Shannon Kliendienst, Manager–Media and Communications, Sydney

Tomoyuki Hamada, Press Relations, Tokyo's Narita Airport

Connie Turner, Communications, Toronto Airport

Vancouver Airport Authority

These gracious people from a wide range of the world's airlines provided a complete array of domestic and international menus from a variety of routes and classes:

Robin Urbanski and the Communications Department, United Airlines

Mike Flanagan, Corporate Communications, American Airlines

Cynthia Schaeffer, Manager, Product Support, Food Services Division, Continental Airlines

Debra Williams and Anne Stephenson, Communications, Air Canada

John Lampl, Vice President, Communications, and Lisa Lam, Communications, British Airways

Jennifer Urbaniak, North America Communications Manager, Lufthansa

Brandon Hamm, Spokesman, JetBlue

Joe Hodas, Spokesman, Frontier Airlines

Delta Airlines Corporate Communications

Chris Malo, Public Affairs, Air France

David Castelveter and Carmen Lugo, Corporate Communications, US Airways

Andrew Christie, Corporate Communications Coordinator, America West

Amanda Tobin, Spokeswoman, Alaska Airlines

Tracy Carlson on behalf of Northwest Airlines

Jennifer Almer, Cohn and Wolfe, for Air New Zealand

Kelly Monks, Communications, Cathay Pacific

Terry Tegesi, Qantas North America

Brandy King, Corporate Communications, Southwest

Keoni Wagner and Patrick Dugan, Communications, Hawaiian Airlines

Communications Department, Singapore Airlines

Laura Bennett for Spirit Airlines

Icelandair North American Communications Department

Caroline Berchtold, Product Communication Manager, SwissAir

Air India North American Communications Department

Tom Fredo, North American Communications, SAS

Carol Anderson, Manager–Public Relations and Advertising, Japan Air

Cruise-line menus were another key component of our research. While easy to obtain, they were not always easy to decipher. So thanks to:

Andy Newman, Carnival/Holland America/Starclubber
Heather Krasnow, Corporate Communications, NCL/Orient
Liz Jakeway, Royal Caribbean/Celebrity
Lyan Sierra-Caro, Royal Caribbean
Julie Benson, Princess Cruises
Mimi Weisband and Crystal Cruises
Rick Meadows, Holland America
Amy Patti, Account Supervisor, NCL

And for providing (or at least pointing us in the correct direction of) fitness and health statistics:

Cassie Piercey, Public Relations, American Council on Exercise
Brooke Correia, Communications, IHRSA

Then, the hotel contingent, who ranged from locations in India to Indonesia, and from Ohio to Botswana:

Wendy Gordon Reisman, former Corporate Director of Food and Beverage Public Relations, The Ritz-Carlton Hotel Company, LLC
Mark Ricci, Starwood
Jamie Izaks, Hyatt
Lisa Caruso at Laura Davidson PR for Marriott
Nicola Blazier, Four Seasons
Vivian Deuschl and Kelly Englehart, Ritz-Carlton
Joan Cronson, Radisson
Darcie Brossart, Wyndham
Lori Armon, Hyatt
Allison Goldstein, Kimpton
Jamie Law, Kimpton
Jennifer Zimmerman, Ramada Inn
Kasey Cavanaugh and Laura Davidson, Marriott/Westin/Sheraton/W/etc.

Caroline Sanphillipo and Carolyn Hergert, InterContinental
Stephanie Yudin, Crown Plaza
Natasha Gullett, Communications, Hotel Indigo/Holiday Inn
Express/Staybridge Suites
Virginia Bush Osborne, Communications, Holiday Inn/Candle-
wood
Jeanne Datz, Communications, Hilton Hotels
The Grand Hyatt, Bangkok, Thailand

And last, but certainly not least, Andy Keown, Communications, Hilton Hotels, for his often-fancy last-minute footwork
for us.

A very special thanks to the entire team at the Physicians
Committee for Responsible Medicine, who performed the analysis of so many food items at airports:

Neal D. Barnard, M.D., Founder and President of the Physicians
Committee for Responsible Medicine
Nutritionists Amber Green and Dulcie Ward
Jeanne McVey, Senior Media Relations Specialist, and Patrick Sul-
livan, Communications Director

And a big thank-you to Cynthia Sass, Registered Dietician
and Spokesperson for the American Dietetic Association, for
doing a major analysis of nearly all nutritional information I collected.

Thanks also to Susan Bowerman, Assistant Director of UCLA
Center for Human Nutrition, for tips about eating on airplanes.

Hotel Chefs:
Lawrence McFadden Vice President, Culinary, and Corporate
Chef, Ritz-Carlton
Jean-Sébastien Kling, Director of Food and Beverage, Europe and
Africa Hilton International

Paul Keeler, Vice President–Food and Beverage, Hilton Hotels Corporation

Dieter Kadoke, Senior Vice President, Food and Beverage, Wyndham

Thomas W. Griffiths, C.M.C., C.H.E., Chef and Professor in Culinary Arts, The Culinary Institute of America

Trainers:
Josh Thurbon, Fitness Director, Celebrity Cruises

Deb Killmon

Monique McDaniel, Personal Trainer, Mytmo Fitness, Kansas City, Missouri

And still more thanks to:

The staff at Nutrax

Dr. James O. Hill at the the University of Colorado at Denver and Health Sciences Center (UCDHSC)

Edmund S. Greenslet, ESG Aviation Services

Peter C. Yesawich, Chairman and CEO, Yesawich, Pepperdine, Brown and Russell

Dave Baurac, Communications and Public Affairs, Argonne National Laboratory. (Dave Baurac developed the software and has the license to sell the diet.)

Bernie Schroeder, Senior Vice President, Marketing and Communications, IDEA Health & Fitness Association, and Kathie Davis, Executive Director and Founder

Lester Robinson, CEO Detroit Airport

Professor Peter Jones, IFCA Chair of Production and Operations Management, University of Surrey, United Kingdom

Dr. Samuel Goldhaber, Professor of Medicine, Harvard Medical School

Meir H. Kryger, M.D., Past President, American Academy of Sleep Medicine; Professor of Medicine, University of Manitoba; Director, Sleep Disorders Centre, St. Boniface Hospital Research Centre, Winnipeg, Manitoba, Canada

Professor Eve Van Cauter, Professor, Department of Medicine Committee on Molecular Metabolism and Nutrition, University of Chicago

Joe McInerney, President, American Hotel and Lodging Association

Steven N. Blair, PED President and CEO, The Cooper Institute, Dallas, Texas

Madelyn H. Fernstrom, Ph.D., Director, UPMC Weight Management Center; Associate Professor of Psychiatry and Surgery, University of Pittsburgh School of Medicine; Associate Professor of Epidemiology, University of Pittsburgh Graduate School of Public Health; Associate Director, UPMC Center for Nutrition

Michael Jacobson, Executive Director, and Jayne Hurley, Nutritionist, Center for Science in the Public Interest. *Thank you!*

Dr. James Levine, endocrinologist at the Mayo Clinic

Charles Czeisler, M.D., Ph.D., Frank Baldino Jr., Ph.D., Professor of Sleep Medicine, Harvard Medical School and Brigham and Women's Hospital

Timothy H. Monk, Ph.D., D.Sc., Professor of Psychiatry, School of Medicine, and Director, Human Chronobiology Program, Western Psychiatric Institute and Clinic

Dixie L. Thompson, Ph.D., Associate Professor, Department of Exercise, Sport, and Leisure Studies; Director, Center for Physical Activity and Health, University of Tennessee

And I—and the folks at Goodwill Industries—thank men's fashion expert Warren Christopher, former Fashion Editorial Director at *Men's Health* magazine, who had the unenviable task of confronting me with all the clothes in my closet that no longer fit or looked good and making me donate all the stuff I stupidly wanted to keep. Warren was really there to remind me not only that did I not fit into those extra-size clothes anymore, but also that I didn't want to fit into those clothes ever again.

And finally, the most special thanks to the most amazing woman, Lyn Benjamin, for reasons only she knows. Without her, this book, and a lot of other wonderful things in my life, would simply not be possible, or even worth it.

Index

ABOUT THE AUTHOR

PETER GREENBERG is the travel editor for NBC's *Today* show. He is also the chief correspondent for the Discovery Network's Travel Channel, editor-at-large of *National Geographic Traveler* magazine, as well as a regular contributor to CNBC and MSNBC. He can be seen often on *The Oprah Winfrey Show*. He lives in Los Angeles, New York, and Bangkok, when he's not living in hotels.